A Guide to Laboratory Investigations

M.F. McGHEE, *MB, BS, MRCS, LRCP, MRCGP, DRCOG*

Radcliffe Medical Press
OXFORD

© 1989 Radcliffe Medical Press Ltd
15 Kings Meadow, Ferry Hinksey Road, Oxford OX2 0DP

British Library Cataloguing in Publication Data

A Guide to Laboratory Investigations
1. Medicine. Laboratory techniques–
Manuals
I. Title
610'.28
ISBN 1 870905 15 6

Photoset by Enset (Photosetting).
Printed in Great Britain by
Billing & Sons Ltd, Worcester

CONTENTS

Preface, v

Acknowledgements, vi

Glossary, vii

Haematology, 1

Red cell indices, 1

Anaemia, 3

White cell indices, 7

Platelets, 10

Blood coagulation tests, 11

Appendix, 14

Biochemistry, 15

Liver function tests, 15

Urea and electrolytes, 23

Urine biochemistry, 26

Blood sugar, 30

Creatine kinase, 33

Lactic dehydrogenase, 34

Thyroid function tests, 35

Blood lipids, 38

Microbiology, 46

Gastrointestinal organisms, 46

Urogenital organisms, 50

Other organisms, 56

Cerebrospinal fluid, 61

Fertility and Pregnancy Testing, 64

Female hormone profiles, 64

Semen analysis, 66

Pregnancy tests, 67

Rhesus blood group testing, 68

Alpha feto proteins, 69

Miscellaneous, 70

Virilism, 70

Interpretation of cervical smears, 71

Microscopic haematuria, 74

Faecal fats, 76

Therapeutic target ranges of commonly monitored drugs, 77

Immunofluorescent autoantibodies, 80

Body mass index, 84

References, 87

Index, 88

PREFACE

This book provides guidelines on interpreting normal and abnormal laboratory results. Many sources of normal values already exist, but not all investigations and their results provide straightforward answers. Interpretation of results is often required and further investigations may have to be considered.

What is the diagnosis, for example, in a patient with an unexpected isolated low platelet count? Thrombocytopenia might initially spring to mind, but what about folate deficiency? Which further investigations do you ask the laboratory to carry out when an isolated raised bilirubin is reported in a healthy individual with normal liver function tests?

In a clear and concise manner this book helps to clarify these and other difficulties that might arise. It is not a substitute for a good history and thorough examination, but acts as a useful adjunct, helping to verify the clinical findings.

I have tried to make the notes accompanying reference values concise. Lists may not be exhaustive but nevertheless important causes of diseases to be considered are always included. As a general practitioner myself, I have included relevant comments and common causes for abnormal values in my own experience. This should not however devalue the text for medical students and hospital doctors.

The normal values and ranges in this book are those familiar to the author. Whilst every effort has been made to check the figures quoted in the text, any errors are my responsibility. If the range of normal values is different from those quoted by a local laboratory then the local results should be regarded as the correct ones. The accompanying notes, however, will still be relevant. The normal range quoted by a laboratory usually includes 95% of a healthy adult population (two standard deviations). Therefore, one in forty results will be higher and one in forty will be lower than this range, i.e. slightly but not markedly outside the normal range. Some test results do not have a normal distribution, gamma GT for example has a non Gaussian type distribution, and these considerations have been taken into account.

M.F. McGHEE
February 1989

v

ACKNOWLEDGEMENTS

My thanks to the many colleagues at the Derby, Nottingham and Leicester hospitals; in particular Dr Deidre Mitchell, Dr Ian Peacock, Dr Richard Powell, Dr Peter Hill, Dr Tony Mellersh, Dr David Bullock, Dr Tony Winder, Dr John Harrop and Mr Ian Scott.

My thanks also to a very patient and forgiving typist Marilyn Wakefield.

GLOSSARY

ACE	Angiotensin Converting Enzyme
AIDS	Acquired Immune Deficiency Syndrome
ALO	Actinomyces Like Organisms
ALT	Alanine Transferase
ANA	Antinuclear Antibodies
ASO	Antistreptolysin-O
AST	Aspartate Transferase
BMI	Body Mass Index
CAD	Coronary Artery Disease
CEA	Corioembryonic Antigen
CHD	Coronary Heart Disease
CIN	Cervical Intraepithelial Neoplasia
CK	Creatine Kinase
CLL	Chronic Lymphatic Leukaemia
CRP	C-reactive Protein
CSF	Cerebrospinal Fluid
CVA	Cerebrovascular Accident
DIC	Disseminated Intravascular Coagulation
DNA	Deoxyribonucleic Acid
DVT	Deep Vein Thrombosis
ECG	Electrocardiograph
ESR	Erythrocyte Sedimentation Rate
FDP	Fibrin Degradation Products
FSH	Follicle Stimulating Hormone
FTA ABS	Fluorescent Treponemal Antibody Absorption Test
FT_4I	Free Thyroxine Index
G-6-PD	Glucose-6-phosphate-dehydrogenase
GFR	Glomerular Filtration Rate
GGT	Gamma Glutamyl Transferase

GIT	Gastrointestinal Tract
GTT	Glucose Tolerance Test
Hb	Haemoglobin
HCG	Human Chorionic Gonadotrophin
HDL	High Density Lipoprotein
HDLC	High Density Lipoprotein Cholesterol
HDN	Haemolytic Disease of the Newborn
HVA	Homovanillic Acid
IDL	Intermediate Density Lipoprotein
IHD	Ischaemic Heart Disease
INR	International Normalised Ratio
IUCD	Intrauterine Contraceptive Device
IVP	Intravenous Pyelogram
KCCT	Kaolin Cephalic Clotting Time
LDH	Lactic Dehydrogenase
LDL	Low Density Lipoprotein
LDLC	Low Density Lipoprotein Cholesterol
LFT	Liver Function Tests
LH	Lutenising Hormone
LUC	Large Unstained Cells
MAOI	Monoamine Oxidase Inhibitor
MCH	Mean Corpuscular Haemoglobin
MCHC	Mean Corpuscular Haemoglobin Concentration
MCV	Mean Corpuscular Volume
MI	Myocardial Infarction
MSU	Midstream Urine Specimen
NSAID	Non Steroidal Anti Inflammatory Drug
OA	Osteoarthritis
OTC	Over The Counter
PA	Pernicious Anaemia
PCV	Packed Cell Volume
PE	Pulmonary Embolism
PID	Pelvic Inflammatory Disease
PRV	Polycythaemia Rubra Vera
PUO	Pyrexia of Unknown Origin
RA	Rheumatoid Arthritis
RAHA	Rheumatoid Arthritis Haemagglutination Assay
RAST	Radio Allergosorbent Test
RBC	Red Blood Cell Count
SLE	Systemic Lupus Erythematosus
T_3	Tri-iodothyronine
T_4	Thyroxine

TB	Tuberculosis
TBG	Thyroxine Binding Globulin
TC	Total Cholesterol
TG	Triglyceride
TIBC	Total Iron Binding Capacity
TOP	Termination of Pregnancy
TPHA	Treponema Pallidum Haemagglutination Assay
TRAb	Thyrotrophin Antibody
TRH	Thyrotrophin Releasing Hormone
TSH	Thyroid Stimulating Hormone
UTI	Urinary Tract Infection
VD	Venereal Disease
VDRL	Venereal Disease Reference Laboratory
VLDL	Very Low Density Lipoprotein
VMA	Vanilmandelic Acid
WBC	White Blood Cell Count
WR	Wassermann Reaction
Ca^+	Calcium
Cl	Chloride
Cu^2	Copper
dl	Decilitre
fl	Femtolitre
g	Gram
H_2O	Water
h	Hour
im	Intramuscular
iu	International unit
iv	Intravenous
K^+	Potassium
kg	Kilogram
l	Litre
Li^+	Lithium
mEq	Milli equivalent
mg	Milligram
Min	Minute
ml	Millilitre
mm^3	Millimetres cubed
mmHg	Millimetres of mercury pressure
mmol	Millimol
Na^+	Sodium
ng	Nanogram
nmol	Nanomol

pg	Picogram
pmol	Picomole
Sec	Second
μ	Micro
μg	Microgram
μmol	Micromol
Zn^2	Zinc

%	Percentage
>	More than
<	Less than
$\geq$	More than or equal to
=	Equals

HAEMATOLOGY

RED CELL INDICES

Haemoglobin (Hb)

- Normal range (g/dl): Adult male: 13.5–18
  Adult female: 11.5–16.5
  Children: at birth: 19±5
  2 weeks: 16
  2 months: 14
  6 months: 11.5–16.5
  puberty male: 13.5–18
  puberty female: 11.5–16

Abnormal test results

- Raised Hb *suggests*:
  Polycythaemia
- Lowered Hb *suggests*:
  Anaemia

Haematocrit or packed cell volume (PCV)

- Normal range (%): Adult male: 40–54
  Adult female: 35–47
- Raised levels indicate increased red blood cell production e.g. chronic hypoxia, polycythaemia rubra vera (PRV) *or* lowered plasma volume e.g. stress polycythaemia or pseudopolycythaemia *NB* Stress polycythaemia can be caused by hypertension, smoking and stress
- PCV consistently > 45 is strongly associated with thromboembolic disease
- Lowered in blood volume loss

Mean corpuscular volume (MCV)

- Normal range (μm^3): 80–99

Mean corpuscular haemoglobin (MCH)

- Normal range (pg): 27–33

Mean corpuscular haemoglobin concentration (MCHC)

- Normal range (g/dl): 32–36

Red blood-cell count (RBC)

- Normal range ($\times 10^6/mm^3$): Adult male: 4.5–6.5
  Adult female: 3.9–5.6

ANAEMIA

- Anaemia with normal white cells and platelets may be:
  hypochromic microcytic
  normochromic normocytic
  or macrocytic

Hypochromic microcytic anaemia

- Caused by:
  Iron deficiency through blood loss or dietary deficiency
  Thalassaemia
  Lead poisoning
  Chronic disorders (occasionally)

Normochromic normocytic anaemia

- Caused by:
  Chronic disorders e.g. renal failure, rheumatoid arthritis (RA)
  Pregnancy
  Haemolysis

Haemolysis

- May be congenital:
  Sickle cell disease
  Thalassaemia
  Congenital spherocytosis
  G-6-PD deficiency causing haemolysis with certain drugs (e.g. sul-
  phonamides, nitrofurantoin, quinine)
- May be acquired:
  Infections e.g. mononucleosis, mycoplasma
  Systemic lupus erythematosus (SLE)
  Drugs e.g. Methyldopa, penicillin, cephalosporin, quinine
  Systemic disease e.g. liver disease, uraemia
  Acute blood loss
  Malignancy

Pancytopenia

- Due to bone marrow failure or premature destruction of the cells and may be due to:
  Malignant disease in the marrow
  Autoimmune disease e.g. RA, SLE
  Increased splenic activity or destruction e.g. portal hypertension
  Aplastic anaemia, which can be due to drugs e.g. antithyroids, antidepressants, anticoagulants, antibiotics, antihistamines, tranquillizers and thiazide diuretics

Macrocytic anaemia

- MCV > 99 which occurs in megaloblastic anaemia

Megaloblastic anaemia

- May be caused by:
  B_{12} deficiency *due to* diet e.g. Hindu vegetarians, vegans
  Post gastrectomy and ileal resection
  Pernicious anaemia (PA) (lack of intrinsic factor)
  Blind loop syndrome
  Fistulae and tapeworms
  Jejunal diverticulosis
  Folate deficiency *due to* drugs e.g. anticonvulsants, trimethoprim, triamterene or poor diet
  Malabsorption
  Pregnancy
  Myxoedema
  Haemolysis (which can be distinguished by polychromasia and raised reticulocyte count)

Serum ferritin

- Normal range (ng/ml): Male: 30–300
                                      Female: 15–150
- Iron protein complex which plays a part in absorption, transport and storage

Abnormal test results

- Low serum ferritin *indicates*:
  Iron deficiency

- Lowered serum ferritin, lowered folate and low B_{12} *suggests*:
  Malabsorption

- Raised ferritin *suggests*:
  Liver disease
  Malignancy
  Chronic inflammatory disease

NB The lower limit of the normal range is lowered in chronic disease e.g. RA with ferritin of 40 is probably iron deficient

Serum iron

- Normal range (μg %): 80–150

Abnormal test results

- Lowered serum iron, lowered total iron binding capacity, with normal or raised ferritin *suggests*:
  Anaemia of chronic disease

- Increased serum iron *seen in*:
  Iron overload
  Contraceptive pill users
  Cirrhosis
  Anaemias e.g. haemolysis

Total iron binding capacity (TIBC)

- Normal range (μmol/l): 45–70

Polycythaemia rubra vera (PRV)

- Characterised by raised Hb, raised white blood cell count (WBC), raised platelets, low MCV and low erythrocyte sedimentation rate (ESR)
- Primary PRV will have raised red cell mass with normal plasma volume
- Secondary PRV occurs secondary to tissue hypoxia in pulmonary disease and congenital heart disease. It will have raised red cell mass with normal WBC and normal platelet count
- Pseudopolycythaemia or stress polycythaemia is characterised by a normal WBC, normal platelet count, normal red cell mass but decreased plasma volume

Serum folate

- Normal range (μg/l): 2–14
- Red cell folate better guide to tissue stores

Red cell folate

- Normal range (μg/l): 130–620
- May be low in B_{12} deficiency states
- May be surprisingly normal during megaloblastic anaemia of pregnancy and after blood transfusion
- For causes of folate deficiency *see* p. 4

Vitamin B_{12}

- Normal range (ng/l): 170–700
- In PA levels often < 50
- 10–15% of people with PA have normal B_{12}

Serum haptoglobin

- Serum protein that combines with Hb
- Normal range (g/l): 0.3–2.0
- Measured principally in patients in whom acute haemolysis is suspected when levels may fall below 0.1
- An increase in haptoglobin occurs in many systemic diseases and inflammatory conditions

WHITE CELL INDICES

White blood-cell count (WBC)

- Normal range ($\times 10^9$/l): 4–11
- Rarely exceeds 50×10^9/l except in leukaemia

NB African normal range is lower

Differential WBC

- Normal range ($\times 10^9$/l): Neutrophils: 2.5–7.5 (60–70%)
  Lymphocytes: 1.5–4.0 (25–30%)
  Monocytes: 0.2–0.8 (5–10%)
  Eosinophils: 0.04–0.44 (1–4%)
  Basophils: up to 0.1 (up to 1%)
- Eosinophils may be elevated in allergies, e.g. eczema, hay fever, or in worm infestations, e.g. schistosomiasis

Abnormal test results

■ Raised WBC, neutrophils > 75% *suggests*:
Bacterial infections

NB Young children normally have a reverse differential

■ Raised WBC, lymphocytes > 45% *suggests*:
Infections, e.g. viral, protozoal, bacterial

NB Such a result is also seen in young children

■ Raised WBC, eosinophils > 6% *suggests*:
Allergic reactions, e.g. to drugs, parasites
Polyarteritis
Reticulosis
Sarcoidosis
Myeloproliferative disorders
Leukaemia

■ Raised WBC (leucocytosis) *commonly found in*:
Pregnancy
Post trauma, e.g. burns, surgery
Post haemorrhage
Malignancy

Drugs, e.g. steroids, digoxin
Myocardial infarction (MI)
Myeloproliferative disease
Renal failure
Gout
Diabetes mellitus
Chronic lymphatic leukaemia (CLL)

■ Lowered WBC (leucopenia), normal Hb, normal platelets *suggests*:
Viral infections
Bacterial infections, e.g. overwhelming septicaemia, brucellosis, miliary tuberculosis
Drugs, e.g. thiouracil
Folate or B_{12} deficiency
Iron deficiency anaemia
Myxoedema thyrotoxicosis
Agranulocytosis (severe leucopaenia in an ill patient)
● Agranulocytosis can be caused by:
Drugs giving rise to pancytopenia e.g. antimitotic drugs and anti-rheumatic drugs such as gold
Some malignancies e.g. leukaemia, non-Hodgkins lymphoma may present with low WBC

Large unstained cells (LUC)

● New parameter included in the automated differential WBC by some laboratories
● Normal range (%): Adults: 0–6
                                   Children: 0–10
● If LUC > 6%, the laboratory will perform a manual differential count

Chronic lymphatic leukaemia (CLL)

● There are 5 stages of CLL:
  0 Lymphocytosis, normal marrow function except increased lymphocytes
  1 Lymphadenopathy in addition to above
  2 Splenomegaly in addition to above
  3–4 Either Hb < 10 or platelets < 100 indicating impaired bone marrow function
● Prognosis is good for patients in stages 0–2 of the disease and poor for patients in stages 3 and 4, about 2–3 years

- Patients in stage 0 do not require treatment; those in stages 1 and 2 require treatment only if there are pressure symptoms from grossly enlarged nodes or spleen

Erythrocyte sedimentation rate (ESR)

- This measurement differs widely in various physiological and pathological conditions
- The 'normal' range varies depending upon the technique e.g. Westergren or seditainer
- Approximate normal range for males = age in years ÷ 2, for females = age in years + 10 ÷ 2

Abnormal test results

■ Raised ESR *suggests*:
Disease
NB Very high (> 100) ESR is found in autoimmune disease, malignancy, acute post trauma and serious infection

■ Low ESR *is found in*:
Heart failure
PRV
Sickle cell anaemia
Treatment with steroids

PLATELETS

- Normal range (10^9/l): 150–400

Abnormal test results

■ Low platelet count *found in*:
Idiopathic thrombocytopenic purpura and other autoimmune disorders
Folate deficiency
Marrow hypoplasia e.g. myelofibrosis and drugs (e.g. sulphonamides, quinine, chlorthiazides and alcohol)

■ Increased platelet count *found in*:
Trauma
Infection and inflammation
Rebound thrombocytosis after haemorrhage, haemolysis, PA, alcoholism or post splenectomy
Malignancy
Chronic inflammatory bowel disease
Essential thrombocythaemia

BLOOD COAGULATION TESTS

- A family and drug history is essential and the following clotting and bleeding time tests may be of help

Skin bleeding times

- Normal range varies with technique, consult laboratory where test performed

Simplate II technique

- Inflate sphygmomanometer to 40 mmHg and make incision 1 mm deep by 5 mm long. Mop blood every 30 sec with cotton wool
- Normal range (min): 2.5–9.5

NB Patient must not have taken aspirin or NSAIDs in previous 10 days

- This test should be carried out as well as a platelet count
- Prolonged test *suggests*:
  Reduced platelets
  Platelets do not function properly
  Von Willebrand's disease but *not* any other clotting defect disorders

NB Platelet dysfunction may be inherited or acquired due to drugs or malignancy

Duke's bleeding time

- Used in the same circumstances as Simplate II technique
- Normal range (min): 2–5

Whole blood clotting time

- Normal range (min): 4–15
- Whole venous blood in a glass tube is mechanically agitated until clotting occurs, this crudely tests the intrinsic clotting mechanism

Plasma fibrinogen

- Normal range (g/l): 1.5–4.0
  (%): 0.2–0.4

Abnormal test results

■ Decreased levels *found in*:
Liver disease
Disseminated intravascular coagulation (DIC)

■ Increased levels *found in*:
Following tissue damage or infection
Pregnancy
Nephrotic syndrome
Collagen disease

Fibrin degradation products (FDP)

● Normal range (mg/l): < 10

Abnormal test results

■ Raised levels *found in*:
Increased fibrinolysis such as post-MI, deep vein thrombosis (DVT), PE
Menstruation
Liver or renal failure

Activated partial thromboplastin time

● Also known as kaolin cephalic clotting time (KCCT)
● Normal range (sec): 43±7
● A measurement of the intrinsic side of the clotting factor cascade

Abnormal test results

■ Prolonged results *occur in*:
Clotting defects, usually factors VIII and IX, occasionally XI and XII
Liver disease
After massive transfusions

Prothrombin time

● Normal range (sec): Control ±4
● Tests the extrinsic clotting system
● The result is inversely proportional to the prothrombin content of the blood tested
● One of the tests used to monitor oral anticoagulants

Thrombin time

- Normal range (sec): Control ±2
- Used for same purpose as prothrombin time

Prothrombin ratio and international normalised ratio (INR)

- International ratio that ensures quality control
- Measures patients prothrombin time compared to the control, used to monitor warfarin and heparin treatment
- Therapeutic range varies according to the condition being treated e.g. simple DVT therapeutic range = 2–3, artificial heart valves and repeated thromboembolism therapeutic range = 3–4

Thrombo test

- Another test to measure warfarin therapy
- Normal range (%): 7–17

Guidance in patients taking warfarin

- Compliance or non-compliance with medication is the commonest cause of unexpected results
- Prothrombin time or ratio, INR and thrombo test may be affected in patients taking warfarin in the following way:
  The action may be inhibited by drugs e.g. carbamazepine, griseofulvin, rifampicin, oral contraceptive pill
  The action may be potentiated in congestive cardiac failure and by drugs e.g. alcohol, allopurinol, cimetidine, cotrimoxazole, danazol, erythromycin, Flagyl, miconazole, sulphonamides and thyroxine
- Any patient requiring very high doses of warfarin to achieve anticoagulation may have a rare inherited condition of resistance to it and requires referral

Thrombophilia

- Inherited or acquired tendency to abnormal clotting
- Consider in people < 40 years with recurrent thromboembolic disease *or* primary thromboembolic event with strong family history
- Check antithrombin III, protein C and protein S
- Refer to haematologist

APPENDIX—SOME COMMON HAEMATOLOGICAL TERMS

Anisocytes

- Abnormal shaped cells sometimes associated with megaloblastic anaemia

Spherocytes

- Abnormally thick red cells associated with hereditary spherocytosis and haemolytic disorders

Target cells

- Associated with iron deficiency, anaemia, haemoglobinopathy including thalassaemia, liver disorders and splenectomy

Hypochromasia

- Taking stain less readily/intensely than usual
- A feature of:
  Iron deficiency
  Thalassaemia
  Lead poisoning
  Sideroblastic anaemia
  Chronic disease

BIOCHEMISTRY

LIVER FUNCTION TESTS (LFT)

Serum bilirubin

- Normal range (μmol/l): < 17
- If bilirubin is elevated with otherwise normal LFT's, ask laboratory to specify level of conjugated/unconjugated bilirubin

Abnormal test results

- Raised level of unconjugated bilirubin *suggests*:
  Gilbert's syndrome *or*
  Haemolysis (can be confirmed by raised reticulocytes > 2%)

- Raised level of conjugated bilirubin *suggests*:
  Liver disease *or*
  Dubin-Johnson syndrome
NB Measurement of conjugated/unconjugated bilirubin not helpful in the differential diagnosis of liver disease

Urinary bile pigments

Abnormal test results

- Raised bilirubin, absent or decreased urobilinogen *suggests*:
  Obstructive jaundice (*see* p. 20)

- Normal or raised bilirubin, normal or raised urobilinogen *suggests*:
  Hepatocellular failure

- Normal bilirubin, raised urobilinogen *suggests*:
  Haemolytic jaundice (*see* p. 20)

Alkaline phosphatase

- Normal range (iu/l): 90–300 (level dependent on method of assay)
- Derived principally from bone, liver, gut and placenta
- In children, levels are 2–3× higher than normal values in adults
- During the pubertal growth spurt, levels may be even higher
- In 3rd trimester of pregnancy, levels are high

- Post menopause levels are raised
- Each individual's level of alkaline phosphatase remains remarkably constant up to 60 years old
- A slightly raised level of alkaline phosphatase is a common laboratory finding; if the test is repeated, and the level continues to rise, further investigation should be performed

Abnormal test results

■ Raised alkaline phosphatase *suggests*:

Bone disease: Osteomalacia and rickets ($Ca^{2+} < 2.12$ mmol/l)
Primary hyperparathyroidism with bone disease ($Ca^{2+} > 2.65$ mmol/l)
Paget's disease of the bone (alkaline phosphatase very high)
Secondary carcinoma of bone (raised Ca^{2+})

or Liver disease: Intra- or extrahepatic cholestasis
Space-occupying lesions (gamma glutamyl transferase (GGT) usually raised but bilirubin may be normal)
Hepatocellular disease

or Hypo- and hyperparathyroidism (*see* p. 28, 29, 36)

Differential diagnosis

- GGT is easily measured, 5-nucleotidase is a more difficult assay
- Measurement of GGT usually sufficient to confirm or exclude hepatic origin of raised alkaline phosphatase

■ Raised alkaline phosphatase, raised GGT *suggests*:
Hepatic origin
- Measurement of 5-nucleotidase (normal range: 3.5–11 iu/l) can confirm or exclude hepatic origin in the presence of isolated raised alkaline phosphatase

■ Raised alkaline phosphatase, raised 5-nucelotidase *suggests*:
Hepatic origin
- Normal 5-nucleotidase excludes hepatic disease

Aspartate aminotransferase (AST) and alanine aminotransferase (ALT)

- Normal range (iu/l): AST: < 50
ALT: < 45

- AST not included in LFT profile in some laboratories
- AST present in high concentrations in heart, liver, skeletal muscle and red blood cells
- ALT present in high concentration in liver; also present in heart and skeletal muscle but in much lower concentrations therefore ALT much more specific to liver disease than AST
- Useful in the differential diagnosis of liver disease
- AST raised in shock, whereas not much elevation of ALT unless liver disease

Abnormal test results

■ Raised levels of ALT:
> 400 iu/l *suggests*:
Acute diffuse hepatocellular damage, e.g. viral hepatitis, toxic damage, ischaemia
> 150 but < 400 iu/l *suggests*:
Chronic, active, protracted, viral or drug induced hepatitis
> 1000 iu/l in jaundice *suggests*:
Acute parenchymal disease
< 100 iu/l in jaundice *suggests*:
Obstructive jaundice

Gamma glutamyl transferase (GGT)

- Normal range (iu/l): Male: up to 51
  Female: up to 33
- Synthesis of GGT stimulated by many drugs, e.g. phenytoin, phenobarbitone, primidone, alcohol, possibly some antidepressants

Abnormal test results

■ Raised GGT, raised MCV *suggests*:
Alcohol abuse (*see* p. 21)

■ Raised GGT, history of excessive alcohol intake, raised ALT and raised MCV *suggests*:
Liver cell damage

- Raised GGT, raised alkaline phosphatase $> 3 \times$ upper limit of normal *suggests*:
  Cholestasis

- Raised GGT *may suggest*:
  Non-specific causes, e.g. MI, cerebrovascular accident (CVA), diabetes mellitus, chronic lung disease[1]

Serum proteins

- Not specific to liver disease
- Not very sensitive
- Normal range (g/l): 60–80, dependent upon method

Albumin

- Normal range (g/l): 30–55, dependant upon method

Abnormal test results

- Elevated albumin (rare) *suggests*:
  Dehydration

- Lowered albumin:
  Check for proteinuria, e.g. nephrotic syndrome, malabsorption, chronic liver disease, pre-eclampsia. Albumin is normally lowered in third trimester
  NB If albumin is reduced, some drugs which are usually protein bound, e.g. phenytoin, phenobarbitone, theophylline, salicylates, penicillin, sulphonamides, warfarin, will be present in higher concentration in their free forms in the bloodstream, therefore toxicity may be apparent at lower drug concentrations

Globulins

- Can be separated by electrophoresis into alpha-, beta- and gamma-globulins
- Normal range (g/dl): Total: 2.0–3.0
                        Alpha-1: 0.2–0.3
                        Alpha-2: 0.4–1.0
                        Beta: 0.6–1.0
                        Gamma: 0.6–1.4

- All gamma-globulins are immunoglobulins; IgG forms 75% of the total

Abnormal test results

- Lowered total globulins *suggests*:
  Immunodeficiency syndromes

- Elevated total globulins *suggests*:
  Paraproteinaemias, e.g. myeloma

- Raised alpha-1 globulin *suggests*:
  Tissue damage
  Oestrogen therapy

- Lowered alpha-1 globulin *suggests*:
  Nephrotic syndrome

- Raised alpha-2 globulin *suggests*:
  Acute inflammatory response
  Nephrotic syndrome (together with lowered albumin and lower gamma globulin)

- Lowered alpha-2 globulin, lowered albumin *suggests*:
  Liver disease
  Malabsorption

- Increased beta-globulin *suggests*:
  Biliary obstruction
  Nephrotic syndrome

- Increased gamma-globulin *suggests*:
  Chronic infection
  RA, also raised alpha-2
  SLE
  Liver disease
  Sarcoidosis

Immunoglobulins

- Normal range: IgA: 1.5–2.5 g/l
  IgG: 8–18 g/l
  IgM: 0.4–2.9 g/l

- Commonly requested in patients presenting with recurrent chest infections or recurrent herpes infections and in children in whom immunodeficiency is suspected
- Immunoglobulins are gamma globulins

Abnormal test results

- Elevated IgM *suggests*:
  Primary biliary cirrhosis
  Chronic infection
  RA
- Antimicrobial antibodies should also be sought in primary biliary cirrhosis

NB IgM is the first immunoglobulin to appear in hepatitis A or B

- Elevated IgA *suggests*:
  Cirrhosis, alcoholic and other forms
  Chronic infection
  Autoimmune disease

- Elevated IgG *suggests*:
  Liver disease
  Autoimmune disease
  Infections

- Decreased IgG *suggests*:
  Nephrotic syndrome

- Homogeneous band of IgG, IgM or IgA on electrophoresis usually *suggests*:
  Myeloma and is usually accompanied by ESR > 100

Bence Jones protein

- Found in the urine of 50% of patients with myeloma
- Also found in other malignant conditions
- A small proportion of patients with myeloma may have Bence Jones protein but *no* elevation of serum proteins
- Does not react with Albustix

Jaundice

- Usually clinically obvious when bilirubin > 35 μmol/l
- The following points in the history may be helpful:

Prodromal flu-like illness *suggests* hepatitis

Sudden onset jaundice with severe pain in otherwise healthy individual *suggests* gallstones

Slow development of jaundice, in the absence of pain or with dull central abdominal pain, anorexia and weight loss *suggests* carcinoma

Previous history of hepatitis *may suggest* chronic active hepatitis

Previous biliary surgery *may suggest* the presence of stones left in the common biliary duct

Previous malignancy, especially of breast or bowel, *may suggest* biliary secondary

Details of alcohol intake should be sought

Members of medical and paramedical professions are at increased risk of contracting viral hepatitis

Foreign travel increases the risks of contracting hepatitis A or B

- Drugs contraindicated and associated with jaundice:
Amitriptyline
Chlorpromazine and other phenothiazines
Chlorpropamide
Erythromycin
Halothane
Imipramine
Indomethacin
Isoniazid
Methyldopa
Phenelzine sulphate and other monoamine oxidase inhibitors (MAOI)
Oral contraceptive pill
Rifampicin
Salicylates
Sulphonamides
Testosterone
Thiouracil

Alcohol abuse

- Alcohol abuse is *suggested by*:
MCV $> 99 \ \mu m^3$ *or* fl
Serum urate $> 520 \ \mu mol/l$
GGT: Male: > 51 iu/l
        Female: > 33 iu/l
AST > 40 iu/l

Triglycerides > 1.8 mmol/l
- Hb: Male: > 18
  - Female: > 16.5
- ALT > 45 iu/l
- Raised gamma-globulins suggest chronic liver disease

Alcohol intoxication (serum volumes), ethanol concentrations

- Subclinical intoxication (g/l): 0–1
- Gross intoxication (g/l): 2
- Stupor (g/l): 3
- Legal limit for blood alcohol whilst driving a motor vehicle = 80 mgm%

UREA AND ELECTROLYTES

Serum values

- Blood samples for electrolytes are best kept at room temperature *but* should be sent to the laboratory within 2 h of collection *or* centrifuged first
- Blood for urea and electrolytes must be placed in correct containers as any contamination even with different bottle lids may cause errors
- Normal range: Na^+: 135–145 mmol/l, 135–145 mEq/l
  K^+: 3.5–5.0 mmol/l, 3.5–5.0 mEq/l
  Cl^-: 95–105 mmol/l, 95–105 mEq/l
  Urea: 3.0–8.8 mmol/l, 8.0–50 mg/100 ml
  Creatinine: 60–120 μmol/l, 0.7–1.4 mg/100 ml
  Bicarbonate 24–32 mmol/l
  Cortisol (9 am) 200–720 μmol/l
  Lead 0.5–1.7 μmol/l
  Cu^{2+}: 16–31 μmol/l, 100–200 μg/100 ml
  Zn^{2+}: 8–23 μmol/l, 0.05–0.15 mg/100 ml

Electrolyte disturbances

- Increased Na^+ *suggests*:
  Primary aldosteronism
  Dehydration

- Decreased Na^+ *suggests*:
  Diarrhoea and vomiting
  Glycosuria
  Heart failure
  Liver failure
  Kidney failure

- Increased K^+ *suggests*:
  Renal failure which can be caused by potassium-sparing diuretics, ACE inhibitors (e.g. captopril), beta-blockers and acidosis
- *Check* that specimen has not been left standing overnight causing haemolysis and leakage from cells of potassium

■ Decreased K^+ *suggests*:
Diarrhoea and vomiting
Diabetes
Drugs e.g. non-potassium-sparing diuretics, steroids, carben-
oxolene, insulin and high-dose penicillin

Urate

● Normal range (μmol/l): Male: < 420
                                            Female: < 360
● Gout likely when uric acid > 600 μmol with normal glomerular fil-
tration rate (GFR), i.e. raised levels expected in renal failure
● Drugs that raise urate levels:
Alcohol
Aspirin (low doses)
Cytotoxic agents
Frusemide
Pyrazinamide
Thiazides
● Dietary constituents that raise urate levels:
Anchovies
Kidney
Liver
Meat extract
Sardines
Shellfish
Turkey
NB Serum urate has been considered a risk factor for ischaemic heart
disease (IHD) but this is no longer considered to be the case

Abnormal test results

■ Decreased urate excretion in urine *occurs in*:
Hypertension
Hypercalcaemia
Myxoedema
Renal failure

■ Increased urate production *occurs in*:
  Haemolysis
  Leukaemia
  Myeloma
  Polycythaemia

Differential diagnosis

- In young patients with marked hyperuricaemia measurement of the 24 h urinary uric acid excretion on a low purine diet identifies stone producers
- Relatives of such patients should be investigated as they are at risk of nephrolithiasis

URINE BIOCHEMISTRY

17 oxosteroids

- Normal range (μmol/24 h): Male 19–50 years: 28–76
  Female 19–50 years: 21–52
  Male > 50 years: 17–63
  Female > 50 years: 10–31

17 oxygenic steroids

- Normal range (μmol/24 h): Male 19–50 years: 28–70
  Female 19–50 years: 21–63
  Male > 50 years: 17–52
  Female > 50 years: 10–31

Abnormal test results

- Elevation of these levels *suggests*:
  Cushing's syndrome
  Polycystic ovaries
  Some testicular cancers
  Adreno-genital syndrome

Vanilmandelic acid (VMA)

- Metabolite of adrenaline and noradrenaline
- Normal range (μmol/24 h): < 45

Abnormal test results

- Raised VMA *suggests*:
  Phaeochromocytoma
  Neuroblastoma

Homovanillic acid (HVA)

- Normal range (μmol/24 h): < 82

EXCRETION OF METABOLITES OVER 24 HOURS

	Mean		Range	
	SI Unit	Traditional Unit	SI Unit	Traditional Unit
Calcium	5.75 mmol	11.5 mEq	3.25–8.25 mmol	6.5–16.5 mEq
Chloride				
Men	184 mmol	184 mEq	120–140 mmol	120–140 mEq
Women	132 mmol	132 mEq		
Creatine	up to 380 mol			up to 50 mg
Creatinine				
Men	15.8 mmol	1.8 g	9.7–23.0 mmol	1.1–2.5 g
Women	10.3 mmol	1.17 g	9.0–11.7 mmol	1.0–1.3 g
Magnesium	5.3 mmol	10.5 mEq	2.5–8.0 mmol	5.0–16 mEq
Nitrogen (total)	0.8 mmol	11.5 g	0.5–1.2 mmol	7–16 g
Oxosteroids				
Men	71 μmol	20.5 mg	59–83 μmol	17–24 mg
Women	49 μmol	14 mg	28–70 μmol	8–20 mg
Phosphate	44 mmol	1.4 g	25–62 mmol	0.8–2.0 g
Potassium				
Men	57 mmol	57 mEq	35–80 mmol	35–80 mEq
Women	47 mmol	47 mEq		
Protein		100 mg		
Sodium				
Men	177 mmol	177 mEq	120–220 mmol	120–220 mEq
Women	128 mmol	128 mEq		
Urate	3.2 mmol	0.5 g	0.5–5.9 mmol	0.1–1.0 g
Urea	342 mmol	20.6 g	209–475 mmol	12.6–28.6 g

Abnormal test results

■ Raised HVA *suggests*:
Phaeochromocytoma
Neuroblastoma

NB Other features of phaeochromocytoma include severe hypertension, mild hyperkalaemia, raised haematocrit, and impaired glucose tolerance, lowered potassium and lowered plasma

Osmolality

● Normal range (mmol/kg): 40–1400

Calcium

● Serum calcium is a balance between calcium absorption and renal excretion, bone resorption and bone mineralisation

Abnormal test results

■ $Ca^{2+} > 2.65$ mmol/l *suggests*:
Hypercalcaemia
● Hypercalcaemia can be due to:
Hyperparathyroidism (phosphate usually < 0.75 mmol/l)
Sarcoidosis
Addison's disease
Metastatic bone disease
Multiple myeloma
Vitamin D excess
Thiazide diuretics

■ $Ca^{2+} < 2.12$ mmol/l *suggests*:
Hypocalcaemia
● Hypocalcaemia can be due to:
Hypoparathyroidism (phosphate raised)
Rickets
Osteomalacia
Chronic renal failure
Malabsorption

Phosphate

- Levels of phosphate are closely linked to those of calcium
- Normal range (mmol/l): 0.8–1.45

Abnormal test results

- Raised phosphate *suggests*:
  Renal failure
  Hypoparathyroidism
  Vitamin D excess

- Lowered phosphate *suggests*:
  Hyperparathyroidism
  Rickets (except in renal failure)
  Vitamin D deficiency
  Renal tubular disease
  Bacterial septicaemia

NB drugs that can lower phosphate levels include aluminium hydroxide, anabolic steroids, oestrogen therapy and intravenous infusions

See also alkaline phosphatase, LFT, p. 15.

Differential diagnosis in bone disease

- Very high alkaline phosphatase, raised Ca^{2+} *suggests*:
  Paget's disease

- Low or normal Ca^{2+}, low phosphate, high alkaline phosphatase *suggests*:
  Rickets
  Osteomalacia

- High Ca^{2+}, low phosphate, possible raised alkaline phosphatase, 'pepperpot' skull on X-ray *suggests*:
  Hyperparathyroidism

NB With osteoporosis there are no biochemical changes

BLOOD SUGAR

- Normal range (mmol/l): Fasting: 3.5–5.5 (may be higher in the elderly) *or* post prandial up to 8
- Use fluoride oxalate tubes for collection only, store specimens in refrigerator if delay in reaching lab

Glucose tolerance test (GTT)

After fasting for at least 12 h, patient is given 50 g anhydrous glucose, equivalent to 380 ml of Lucozade. Blood is sampled a half hour before and 1 and 2 h after ingestion of the glucose. Urine is also collected before ingestion and at hourly intervals afterwards.

- Normal (mmol/l): Fasting range: 3–6
  Peak at 0.5–1 h: < 10
  At 2 h: 3–6

Abnormal test results

- Fasting glucose < 8, 2 h glucose > 8 but < 11 *suggests*:
  Impaired glucose tolerance
  Check blood lipids in these patients

- Fasting glucose > 8, 2 h glucose > 11 *confirms*:
  Diabetes mellitus

Note All figures quoted are for plasma; whole blood glucose figures are 15% lower

Confirmation of diabetes mellitus

Diagnosis is confirmed:
- In a patient *with* symptoms with a random glucose > 11, if in doubt perform GTT

Indications for GTT

- Glycosuria but normal blood glucose with or without symptoms
- During pregnancy

Causes of hypo- and hyperglycaemia

- Other causes of hyperglycaemia
  Acromegaly
  Cushing's syndrome
  Pancreatitis
  Phaeochromocytoma
  Thyrotoxicosis
- Drugs which can cause hyperglycaemia
  Thiazide diuretics, especially in combination with anti-hypertensives
  Caffeine
  Chlorpromazine
  Dexamethasone
  Hydrocortisone
  Oral contraceptives
  Nicotine
  Phenytoin
  Prednisolone
  Probenecid
  Warfarin
- Causes of hypoglycaemia
  Liver failure
  Pancreative cell hyperplasia
  Postgastrectomy dumping syndrome
  Renal failure
  Insulinoma
- Drugs which can cause hypoglycaemia
  Alcohol
  Aspirin, barbiturates, beta-blockers
  Chlorpropamide
  Glibenclamide
  Insulin (overdose)
  MAOIs, sulphonamides

Monitoring long-term control of diabetes

HbA$_1$ (%)

- Guidelines:
  Overtreatment: < 6

Very good control: 6–8
Good control: 8–9.5
Increased therapy needed: 9.5–12
Careful monitoring and change of therapy: > 12
NB Local figures for these guidelines should be sought

Serum fructosamine (mmol/l)

- Use of fructosamine assay has replaced that of HbA_1 in monitoring the control of diabetes because it is less expensive, more precise and reflects average blood glucose levels over the preceding 2 weeks
- Guidelines for adult diabetics:
  Good control: < 3.0
  Control could be improved: 3.0–3.7
  Poor control: > 3.7

NB These ranges are correct only when albumin concentration is normal (30–45 g/l). Figures will vary in individual labs

CREATINE KINASE (CK)

- The most sensitive enzymatic detector of acute MI in routine use
- Three isoenzymes of CK exist—MM, BB, MB, MM and MB are present in cardiac muscle
- Normal range (iu/l): Male: 24–195
                         Female: 24–170
- CKMB is expressed as % of total CK

Abnormal test results

- Elevated CK
  Ask lab for CKMB

- > 6% CKMB *suggests*:
  MI
  Request lactic dehydrogenase (LDH) if patient presents with chest pain after 36 h normal (100–500 iu/l). Increased in venous stasis

Differential diagnosis

- Normal CK 12–36 h after onset of chest pain *excludes* MI
- 2 normal CKs (1 taken 12–36 h after onset of symptoms) *excludes* MI
- Raised CK, raised CKMB ratio *confirms* MI
- Raised total CK and CKMB ratio < 5% *can indicate* skeletal or cardiac muscle damage

LACTIC DEHYDROGENASE (LDH)

- Enzymatic detector of acute MI
- Five isoenzymes exist; heart principally contains LDH_1 liver and skeletal muscle contain primarily LDH_4 and LDH_5
- Normal range (iu/l): 100–500

Abnormal test results

■ Elevated LDH *suggests*:
  Acute MI
NB False-positive elevations (< 5% of results) occur in haemolysis, megaloblastic anaemia, leukaemia, liver disease, hepatic congestion, renal disease, some neoplasms, pulmonary embolism, myocarditis, skeletal muscle disease and shock

THYROID FUNCTION TESTS

- Normal range (serum values): Total thyroxine (T_4): 60–135 nmol/l
  Tri-iodothyronine (T_3):
  1.1–2.8 nmol/l
  Serum free T_4: 8.8–23.2 pmol/l
  Serum free T_3: 3.0–8.6 pmol/l
  Thyroxine binding globulin
  (TBG): 8–15 mg/l
  T_4/TBG ratio: 6:12
  Thyroid stimulating hormone
  (TSH): 0.5–5.5 miu/l

Free thyroxine index (FT₄I)

- Normal range: 3.41–5.89, although different methods can cause variation
- Not so commonly used
- Superceded by T_4/TBG ratio

Abnormal test results

- Raised serum T_4 *occurs in*:
  Thyrotoxicosis
  Oestrogen therapy and during pregnancy
  Thyroxine therapy
  Liver disease
  Porphyria
  Familial TBG excess

- Lowered serum T_4 *occurs in*:
  Myxoedema
  Nephrotic syndrome
  Hepatic failure (due to lowered serum albumin)
  Kidney failure
  Congenital TBG deficiency
  Hypopituitarism
  Drugs e.g. phenytoin, NSAIDs

- Low TSH *suggests*:
  Thyrotoxicosis
  Overtreatment with thyroxine

■ Raised TSH *suggests*:
Myxoedema
Undertreatment with thyroxine

■ Lowered T_4, raised TSH and lowered T_4/TBG ratio *suggests*:
Myxoedema
Check for thyroid antibodies

■ Raised T_4, raised T_3, lowered TSH *suggests*:
Thyrotoxicosis
● If result marginal *repeat* tests in 3 months
NB When treating thyrotoxicosis with radioactive iodine the effect is not seen until 6 weeks later. After treatment with radioactive iodine myxoedema will always follow

Differential diagnosis

1 Thyroid releasing hormone (TRH) stimulation test can be used to determine thyroid function in borderline cases
● Normal TSH response to TRH *excludes* hyperthyroidism
● No TSH response to TRH *suggests* hyperthyroidism
● Exaggerated TSH response to TRH *suggests* hypothyroidism
● This test has been superceded by TSH assays

2 Thyrotrophin antibody (TRAb) test can be used to differentiate between Grave's disease and any other cause of hyperthyroidism
● TRAb are equivalent to TSH receptor antibodies
● 50–80% of patients with Grave's disease have raised TRAb
● TRAb > 10 *confirms* Grave's disease
● TRAb < 10 *does not exclude* Grave's disease
● This test is used in few labs

Haemagglutination tests for thyroid antibodies

● Normal range: Microsome titre: up to 800
Colloid titre: up to 800 (also known as thyro-globulm antibodies)

Abnormal test results

- > 1600 *suggests*:
  Autoimmune disease e.g. Hashimoto's disease (levels often very high)
  Grave's disease
  Simple myxoedema

BLOOD LIPIDS[2,3]

- The major plasma lipids are:
  Cholesterol
  Cholesterol ester
  Triglyceride
  Phospholipid
- Lipids and apolipoproteins circulate in the form of macro-molecular complexes known as lipoproteins
- There are 5 major groups of lipoproteins:
  Chylomicrons
  Very low-density lipoprotein (VLDL)
  Low-density lipoprotein (LDL)
  Intermediate-density lipoprotein (IDL)
  High-density lipoprotein (HDL)
- Normal range (mmol/l): Total cholesterol (TC): < 6.5
  LDL: < 3.35
  HDL: Male: 0.9–1.6
  Female: 1.2–2.8
  HDL cholesterol should be ⩾20% of TC
  Triglyceride (TG): < 2.5
  TC/HDL ratio: < 4.5
- The level of total cholesterol recommended by British Hyper-lipidaemia Association: 5.2 mmol/l (about 80% of UK adults have total cholesterol levels > 5.2 mmol/l)
- Optimal levels of total cholesterol may vary with age and sex of individual:
  15–29 years: Male: < 6
  Female: < 6.5
  30–60 years: Male: < 6.5
  Female: < 7
  60+ years: Male: < 7
  Female: < 7
- LDL increases with age; HDL remains constant
- High level of LDL risk factor of IHD; high level of HDL thought to be cardioprotective
- Blood lipids can be altered after any acute illness including MI and should not therefore be measured until three months after the event
- Females with raised cholesterol are hypothyroid until proven otherwise
- Males with raised cholesterol drink excess alcohol until proven otherwise

Sampling

- Blood need not be taken in 'fasting' state, a random sample is sufficient
- Sample should be taken after removal of the tourniquet
- If TC > 6.5 mmol/l
  Take sample in 'fasting' state
  Request triglycerides and HDL

Test results

- TC > 6.5 mmol/l *suggests*:
  Hypercholesterolaemia—significant risk factor for IHD/CAD
NB Hypercholesterolaemia may be *secondary* to:
  - Diabetes mellitus
  - Excess alcohol intake
  - Hypothyroidism (especially in elderly females)
  - Biliary obstruction
  - Chronic renal failure
  - Hypotension
  - Nephrotic syndrome
  - Obesity
  - Pregnancy
  - Therapy with some beta-blockers, steroids, thiazide diuretics, isotretinoin and psoriatic drugs e.g. Tigason
- 70% of hyperlipidaemia due to one of above primary disorders

General Principles of Treatment of hypercholesterolaemia

- The primary aim is to reduce lipid levels to those that are acceptable
- Other risk factors for IHD should also be eradicated e.g. smoking, obesity, excess alcohol, hypertension

Treatment Groups

1 Total cholesterol 5.2–6.5 mmol/l, triglycerides < 2.2 mmol/l
- Lipid-lowering diet
- Weight control
- Drugs rarely necessary
- Follow-up: at 6 months if other risk factors for IHD present; otherwise optional

- No improvement: *Reinforce* dietary advice
  Consider drug therapy

2 Total cholesterol 6.5–7.8 mmol/l, triglycerides < 2.2 mmol/l
- Lipid-lowering diet
- Weight control
- Follow-up: at 2–4 months
- No improvement: *Reinforce* dietary advice
  Consider drug therapy

3 Total cholesterol < 5.2 mmol/l, triglycerides 2.3–5.6 mmol/l
- Lipid-lowering diet
- Weight control
- Drug therapy
- Follow-up: at 12 months; *assess* efficacy of drugs
- No improvement: *Reinforce* dietary advice
  Reassess in 6 months if other risk factors for
  IHD present
- Improvement: *Reassess* in 1–5 years

4 Total cholesterol 5.2–7.8 mmol/l, triglycerides 2.3–5.6 mmol/l
- Lipid-lowering diet
- Weight control
- Follow-up: at 2–4 months
- No improvement: *Give* drug therapy

5 Rare lipid disorders, often of genetic origin, which require precise
  diagnosis and treatment at a lipid clinic

Dietary advice

- Reduce calorie intake to achieve weight control (*see* table on page 84)
- Replace saturated fats with poly- and monounsaturated fats
- Increase intake of fresh vegetables, fruit, wholemeal bread, fibre,
  oats and pulses
- *Consider* referral to dietician

NB Individuals at low risk of IHD will increase their life-expectancy
by 3 months. Individuals at high risk of IHD will increase their life
expectancy by 12 months

Drug therapy

- Drugs that lower lipid levels may be considered in:
  Subjects with known vascular disease, when diet alone has failed
  Subjects with familial hypercholesterolaemia
  Subjects with family history of IHD/CAD
  Subjects whose cholesterol > 7.8 mmol/l
- Agents include:
  Bezafibrate
  Cholestyramine
  Gemfibrozil
  Maxepa
  Zocor (new inhibitor of cholesterol synthesis)
- Maxepa decreases total cholesterol in some patients, decreases trig-
  lycerides, raises HDL

NB Stopping smoking and control of blood pressure will increase a
patient's life-expectancy to a greater degree than lowering total
cholesterol levels

Rare lipid disorders

Familial hypercholesterolaemia

- There are two forms of this inherited condition:
  Heterozygous familial hypercholesterolaemia
  Homozygous familial hypercholesterolaemia (very rare)
- Features:
  Total cholesterol > 6.7 mmol/l, sometimes > 9 mmol/l
  LDL elevated 2–10×normal
  Normal triglyceride levels
  Tendon xanthomas about the knee, elbow and the dorsum of the
  hand
  Xanthelasma
  Corneal arcus
  Family history of early coronary heart disease (CHD) and MI or
  xanthomas
- Treatment:
  Lipid-lowering diet
  Limit other risk factors
  Drug therapy, e.g. Questran, Zocor
  Plasma exchange

Familial triglyceridaemia

- Features (not usually exhibited until puberty/early adulthood):
  Triglyceride levels > 2.5 mmol/l
  VLDL elevated
- Affected individuals frequently have:
  Obesity
  Hyperglycaemia
  Hyperinsulinaemia
  Hypertension
  Hyperuricaemia
- If level of chylomicrons is increased, pancreatitis may develop
- Treatment:
  Control obesity
  Restrict calories, saturated fat and alcohol intake
  Avoid oral contraceptives
  Treat diabetes mellitus and hypothyroidism if present
  If all these measures fail, consider drug therapy, e.g. Maxepa

Familial combined hyperlipidaemia

- Features:
  Elevation in total cholesterol and triglyceride levels from puberty onwards
  Lipid elevations often mild and can change with time
  Strong family history of premature CAD
  Xanthomas absent
- Treatment:
  Weight reduction
  Lipid-lowering diet
  Avoid alcohol
  Avoid oral contraceptives
  Limit other risk factors
  If there is elevation in triglyceride levels, give Maxepa

NB Lowering the level of cholesterol pharmacologically may increase the triglyceride level thereby negating any benefit obtained by this manoeuvre

Familial dysbetalipoproteinaemia

- Features:
  Total cholesterol levels elevated

Triglyceride levels elevated
Xanthomas of palms and digital creases
Tuberous or tuberoeruptive xanthomas over the elbows and knees
Xanthelasma
Corneal arcus

NB Clinical features not usually manifest until affected individual > 20 years

- Patients with clinical manifestations of this condition often have:
  Diabetes mellitus
  Hypothyroidism
  Obesity
- Affected individuals at high risk of IHD and peripheral vascular disease manifest mainly as claudication
- Treatment:
  Treat hypothyroidism and diabetes mellitus if present
  Control obesity
  Lipid-lowering diet
  Limit other risk factors
  If all these measures fail, consider drug therapy, e.g. Bezalip

Classification of hyperlipoproteinaemia

- System based on laboratory definitions

Type I

- Cholesterol normal
- Triglycerides greatly increased
- Hyperchylomicronaemia

Type IIa

- Cholesterol increased
- LDL increased
- Triglycerides normal

Type IIb

- Cholesterol increased
- VLDL increased
- Triglycerides increased
- LDL increased

Type III

- Cholesterol increased
- Triglycerides increased
- VLDL cholesterol/VLDL triglyceride > 0.35
- Floating betalipoproteins

Type IV

- Cholesterol normal or increased
- VLDL increased
- Triglycerides increased

Type V

- Cholesterol increased
- LDL reduced
- Chylomicrons and VLDL increased
- Triglycerides greatly increased

Appropriate drug therapy (where diet alone has failed)

- Type IIa: Cholestyramine
- Type IIb: Bezafibrate
                   Gemfibrozil
- Type III: Bezafibrate
                   Gemfibrozil
- Type IV: Bezafibrate
                   Gemfibrozil
- Type V: Maxepa

Drugs which may adversely affect blood lipids

Some diuretics
Some beta-blockers
Norgestrel containing oral contraceptives
Isotretinoin (treatment of acne)
Tigason (treatment of psoriasis)

LIPOPROTEIN PHENOTYPES AND THEIR MANAGEMENT

Phenotype	Type	Total Cholesterol	LDLC	HDLC	Triglycerides	Treatment
IIa	hyper-cholesterolaemia	raised	raised	raised, normal or low	normal	diet drugs: cholestyramine, bezafibrate, gemfibrozil
IIb	hyper-cholesterolaemia	raised	raised	raised, normal or low	raised	diet drugs: cholestyramine, bezafibrate, gemfibrozil
I, III and IV	combined hypercholesterolaemia and dysbeta-lipoproteinaemia	raised or normal	normal	raised, normal or low	raised	diet drugs: bezafibrate, gemfibrozil
V	hyper-triglyceridaemia	normal		low or normal	raised	diet reduce alcohol if appropriate drugs: Maxepa

Blood lipids can be centrifuged into:
LDLC
HDLC
Elevation of LDLC increases the risks of CHD
HDLC levels are inversely related

MICROBIOLOGY

GASTROINTESTINAL ORGANISMS

- All infectious diarrhoea is notifiable as dysentery or food poisoning to the Department of Environmental Health in order to locate and eradicate the source
- Of particular importance in food handlers in institutions and hospitals

Salmonella

Transmission

- Mainly from food, occasionally from person to person

Treatment

- Ill or toxic patients require admission to infectious diseases hospital
- Patients require supportive treatment only, i.e. fluids

NB Treatment with antibiotics can enhance the incidence of a carrier state

Widal test

- Serological test for typhoid
- Can be helpful in diagnosis of enteric fever but difficult to interpret
- Normal range: *S. paratyphi* A and C: up to 1:10
                  S. typhi and *S. paratyphi* B:
                  H titres up to 1:30
                  O titres up to 1:50
- High titres indicate infection
- Stool culture more helpful than serology

Shigella

Transmission

- Flies, fingers, food and faeces

Presentation

- Same symptoms as Salmonella
- Occasionally patient can become unwell or toxic

Treatment

- If patient is unwell symptomatic treatment should be used
- Septrin is rarely indicated

Giardia lamblia

- Common intestinal protozoan
- May be found in stools of patients especially if they have recently returned from abroad having contracted persistent diarrhoea

Transmission

- Mainly from contaminated water

Presentation

- Fatty, offensive and persistent diarrhoea

Treatment

- Flagyl 2 g daily for 3 days

Campylobacter jejuni

- Commonest cause of bacterial diarrhoea

Transmission

- Person to person is rare
- Not particularly transmissible in food handlers but any food handler with diarrhoea should be excluded from work
- Campylobacter lies in the gut and carcass of chickens and can be spread during their preparation

Presentation

- Fever, diarrhoea and vomiting for up to 2 weeks
- Severe abdominal cramps

Treatment

- Rarely needs treatment
- Erythromycin may be used especially if patient is immunosuppressed or there are severe abdominal cramps

Campylobactor pylori

- Can be eradicated with ampicillin and bismuth chelate (De–Nol)
- Associated with chronic gastritis and relapsing duodenal ulcers

Cryptosporidia

- Organism has become more prevalent since the appearance of AIDS but does occur in others
- Mode of transmission uncertain, possibly zoonosis

Presentation

- Self-limiting gastroenteritis in normal individuals
- Life-threatening diarrhoea in immunologically depressed individuals

Treatment

- No effective treatment

Ascaris (nematode)

- In man, parasite of small intestine

Transmission

- Faeco-oral spread
- Larvae may migrate to lungs (Loeffler's syndrome), intestine and urinary tract

Presentation

- Commonly presented by mother to doctor, may be presented with an earthworm
- Eggs or roundworm in stool
- Blood eosinophilia

Treatment

- Adults and children > 6 years, Pripsen 1 sachet followed by Vermox
- Deworm pets

Enterobius vermicularis (threadworm)

- Commonest intestinal parasite in white patients

Transmission

- Faeco-oral spread

Presentation

- Eggs infrequently found in stools
- Eggs found on perianal skin after placing Sellotape over it
- Intense itching as worms migrate outside anus at night
- Possible appendicitis
- Eosinophilia may be found

Treatment

- Pripsen (as above dosage), repeat after 14 days
- Whole family should be treated as well as affected individual
- Cut children's nails

NB Special care should be taken when changing bed linen

UROGENITAL ORGANISMS

- Refer to genitourinary clinic, many organisms may be present

Herpes genitalis

- Common cause of genital ulceration

Presentation

- In men erythematous red area develops, usually on prepuce, followed by vesicles
- In women commonest sites of vesicles are labia majora and minora, cervix and perineum

Diagnosis

- Confirmed by sending material from ulcer in virus transport medium to lab for culture
- Differential diagnosis includes primary chancre of syphilis, secondary infection after scratching scabies lesions, trauma secondary to sexual intercourse

Treatment

- Analgesics for pain relief
- Zovirax cream 5% and oral Zovirax 200 mg×5 od for 5 days
- In frequently recurrent herpes prophylaxis with oral Zovirax 200 mg 1–4× daily

Gonorrhoea

- 60% of affected women are asymptomatic
- Dysuria in a young man with a normal urinary tract is more likely to have urethritis than urinary tract infection (UTI)

Presentation

- In men discomfort in urethra followed by creamy thick yellow-green purulent discharge
- In women vaginal discharge, dysuria, frequency of micturition, backache or abdominal pain
- Trichomonas also present in 50%

Diagnosis

- In men, swab of urethral discharge should be sent for staining and microscopic examination, and culture
- In women, swab from urethra and cervix should be sent for culture
- Swabs should be transported in Stuart's medium in a bottle with a screw-top

Complement fixation tests (blood test)

- Rarely used and of little value
- Negative in the early stages
- If treatment given soon after diagnosis it never becomes positive
- The longer the infection persists the more likely the test is to remain positive
- If test is positive further clinical examination and swabs are indicated

Treatment

- Seek advice from genitourinary clinic
- Single dose 2.4 mega units procaine penicillin or 3 g ampicillin or 3 g amoxycillin in a single dose, each with probenecid 2 g orally[4]
- For patients allergic to penicillin or where there is a high incidence (> 5%) of penicillinase-producing *Neisseria gonorrhoea* treat with spectinomycin 2 g im or kanamycin 2 g im
- Single dose ciprofloxacin may be effective

Trichomonas vaginalis

- Microscopic parasite
- May be an incidental finding on cervical smear
- May occur in association with other venereal diseases
- Infection can be asymptomatic

Presentation

- In men, urethra or its extensions may be infected and cause reinfection of partner
- In women, frothy vaginal discharge with vaginal tenderness, swollen and inflamed vulva and pain on urination

Diagnosis

- Diagnosis must be made before any treatment is given
- Mix discharge from vagina with warm saline solution and examine under microscope to see parasites
- Can be cultured

Treatment

- If symptomatic Flagyl 200 mg tid × 1 week or 2 g single dose

Gardnerella vaginalis (previously known as Haemophilus vaginalis)

- Bacteria inhabiting vagina whose increased growth in association with that of anaerobic bacteria causes discharge

Presentation

- In women, smelly greyish irritant vaginal discharge
- Fishy smelling odour

Diagnosis

- Found on high vaginal swabs
- Clue cells can indicate possibility of *Gardneralla*

Treatment

- Flagyl 400 mg bd patient and partner × 7 days or 2 g single dose
- May be an antabuse effect with Flagyl
- If discharge is asymptomatic then encourage hygiene

Chlamydia

- Most common cause worldwide of non-gonococcal urethritis in men
- In women the cervix is infected; the infection may be eliminated, may be asymptomatic or can spread to other genital organs to cause pelvic inflammatory disease (PID). As common as gonococcus

Presentation

- In men, mucopurulent urethral discharge and pain on urination, which may be severe; in some cases, there is a frequent need to pass urine and bladder pain
- In women in whom the infection has spread, the patient is ill with fever, and has a painful and tender abdomen
- In neonates red eye and mucopus in the presence of 'cobblestone' appearance of the conjunctival epithelium

Diagnosis

- Endocervical and urethral swab for culture in chlamydia (not viral) transport medium
- In men, discharge can be examined under microscope; sediment from urine sample can be examined microscopically after centrifugation; sample of discharge can be sent for culture
- In neonates, pus should be removed and underlying cells, e.g. conjunctival, sent for culture

Treatment

- Oxytetracycline, doxycycline or minocycline plus metronidazole for women
- Erythromycin 500 mg qd×7–14 days is suitable for pregnant or lactating women

Actinomyces like organisms (ALO)

- Reported in women who have had an intrauterine contraceptive device (IUCD) for many years
- ALO presence is related to length of use of IUCD: after 1 year 1–2% smears contain ALO; after 3 years 8–10%; after 5 years 20%
- Can be asymptomatic

Presentation

- Most commonly asymptomatic
- Pain, dyspareunia, excessive discharge

Treatment

- If *symptomatic*: IUCD to be removed and sent to lab with endocervical swab for culture; if symptoms persist refer to gynaecologist for IUCD removal
- If *asymptomatic*: continue with coil and advise to return if specific symptoms arise. Repeat smear as per routine
  or: remove coil and replace with copper one. Repeat smear in 3–12 months
  or: leave coil and treat with penicillin. Repeat smear after course of treatment
- Where ALO's continue to be reported in an asymptomatic patient an alternative form of contraception should be sought where possible

Syphilis

- Caused by *Treponema pallidum*, the spirochaete
- There are three stages of this disease—primary, secondary, tertiary; the tertiary stage is now rarely seen
- All suspected cases should be referred

Presentation

- In primary syphilis, a hard-edged ulcer, known as a chancre, is seen on the man's penis or women's vulva; lymph nodes in groin may be swollen
- In secondary syphilis, affected individual feels ill and may have headaches and joint pains; there is a pale skin rash which persists for 6 weeks then fades slowly; a few subjects develop ulcers in the mouth, vulva or anus

Diagnosis

- Refer to genitourinary clinic where possible
- Sample of clear fluid taken from the centre of a cleaned chancre is examined under the microscope to detect treponemas
- Blood tests for syphilis are negative for about 6 weeks after infection
- If Venereal Disease Reference Laboratory (VDRL) or treponema pallidum haemagglutination (TPHA) test is positive, the FTA ABS test is used to confirm the diagnosis

- False positives on VDRL may occur after typhoid or yellow fever immunisation, autoimmune disease (RA and SLE) and in other treponemal infections e.g. yaws
- TPHA test can be used instead of VDRL

Treatment

- Penicillin
- Follow-up blood tests for 12 months after treatment essential

NB If neither primary nor secondary syphilis is treated, tertiary syphilis may develop 2–20 years after infection; this is a serious condition which carries a high risk of dying at an early age and is characterised by damage to many different tissues

OTHER ORGANISMS

Toxoplasma

- Protozoal parasite, *Toxoplasma gondii*
- In most cases, affected individuals are asymptomatic or have only subclinical or mild infection
- Unsuspected infection in pregnancy can be passed from mother to unborn child in up to 50% of cases
- Increasing importance in immunocompromised individuals

Presentation

- In the acute illness pneumonia with fever, cough, generalised aches and pains, malaise, maculopapular rash, lymphadenopathy with lymphocytosis showing atypical mononuclear cells similar to those in glandular fever
- Rarely jaundice and myocarditis
- Can cause choroidoretinitis and uveitis in adults
- Infection passed to child *in utero* can cause encephalomyelitis, hydrocephalus, microcephaly, cerebral calcification, choroidoretinitis
- May present with prolonged malaise and has been associated with myalgic encephalomyelitis

Diagnosis

- Antibodies detectable by fluoresence or dye test appear early in disease and persist for years
- Complement fixing antibodies are late to appear and decline more quickly
- 20–40% of normal adults give positive Latex test at titres of 1/8–1/128
- Titre of 1/256 can be expected in 1% of adults
- Any titre, however low, should be seen as indicating infection sometime in the past
- Negative results are uncommon and therefore useful in excluding the disease
- Antibodies may not be detectable in ocular toxoplasmosis
- In ocular toxoplasmosis some cases may give titres of $\geq 1/256$ but majority are 1/8–1/128
- In pregnancy IgM determination can be useful to detect recent infection

Treatment

- Usually only treated in immunosuppressed individuals
- Sulphonamide 1 g qd and pyrimethamine 25 mg daily×2 weeks in all active cases
- Supplements of folic acid are required
- Tetracycline 250 mg qd×4 weeks if this fails
- For uveitis and choroidoretinitis use corticosteroids
- Clindamycin is a newer alternative

Branhamella catarrhalis

- Only of importance in immunocompromised individuals
- Increasingly seen as significant indirect pathogen in respiratory tract infections because it produces beta-lactamase which causes penicillin resistance in other respiratory tract pathogens e.g. *Streptococcus pyogenes*
- Comprises 10% of all isolates from respiratory tract
- More common in mining communities and people with damaged lungs

Treatment

- Penicillins resistant to beta-lactamase production e.g. cloxacillin, flucloxacillin and augmentin
- Seek advice from local laboratory

Pneumocystis carinii

- Pneumonia is becoming more common as opportunistic infection in AIDS patients
- Requires hospital management

Treatment

- Refer to specialist
- High dose co-trimoxazole (trimethoprim 20 mg/kg/day) plus sulphamethoxazole 100 mg/kg/day in divided doses
- A rash can often occur with this treatment but is not a contraindication
- If neutropenia occurs the sulphamethoxazole dosage should be halved or substituted with Dapsone 100 mgm/day

- Alternative treatment is iv Pentamidine 4 mg/kg/day×21 days but only available on a named patient basis
- Maintenance therapy is with low dose co-trimoxazole (trimethoptrim 160 mg/day plus sulphamethoxazole 800 mg/day) or sulphadoxine pyrimethamine (Fansidar) orally 1–2 tablets/week or iv Pentamidine 4 mg/kg fortnightly may prevent relapse

Streptococcus

- Normal range < 200 iu/m

Diagnosis

- Antistreptolysin-O (ASO) titre can confirm infection with streptococcus 2–6 weeks after the organism may have disappeared
- ASO titre should be requested in any condition in which streptococcus is thought to be responsible for the illness, e.g. glomerulonephritis, rheumatic fever, erythema nodosum, Stevens–Johnson syndrome
- Titres > 200 iu/ml *indicate* possible recent streptococcal illness
- It is ideal to detect a rise in titres over 2 tests separated by an interval of 2 weeks
- A rise in titres, e.g. from 100 to 200 iu/ml, *indicates* recent streptococcal illness

NB Several other Gram-positive organisms may cause similar rises in titres

Meningococcal meningitis

- Common in children and young adults

Presentation

- Those of meningitis
- Also purpuric (non-blanching) rash

Treatment

- If suspected, im benzyl penicillin should be given as soon as possible, i.e. before transfer to hospital
- Prophylaxis for relatives are organised by the hospital, usually rifampicin for 48 h

Urine

- Criteria for UTI $= > 10^5$ organisms/ml
- > 100 White cells with no organisms *consider*:
  Venereal disease (VD)
  Malignancy
  Tuberculosis (TB)
  Post irradiation
  Kidney stones

NB Catheter infections rarely require treatment

CEREBROSPINAL FLUID

	Pressure	Gross appearance	Cells ×10^6/l	Protein		Globulin test	Chlorides as NaCl		Glucose		Lange curve	W.R.
				g/l	mg/100 ml		mmol/l	mg/100 ml	mmol/l	mg/100 ml		
Normal	80–200 mm CSF	clear colourless	0–8	0.1–0.45	10–45	neg	120–128	700–750	2.5–4.7	45–85	—	—
Pyogenic meningitis	increased	turbid or purulent	1000–2000+ (Poly-morphs.)	0.5–5.0	50–500	positive	111–120	850–700	0–2.5	0–45	'meningitic'	—
Tuberculous meningitis	increased	clear cobweb clot	100–300 (mostly lymph.)	0.5–1.0	50–100	usually pos	86–103	500–600	0.8–2.5	15–45	sometimes 'meningitic'	—
Acute aseptic meningitis	increased	clear or cloudy	50–1500 (lymph.)	increased	increased	pos	normal	normal	normal	normal	—	—
Poliomyelitis	increased	clear	50–250 (Poly. then lymph.)	0.5–2.0	50–200	pos	normal	normal	normal	normal	—	—
Subarachnoid haemorrhage	increased	bloody xanthochromic	Increased (lymph)	0.5–1.0	50–100	—	—	—	—	—	—	—

CEREBROSPINAL FLUID (CSF)

- Normal range (mm^3): < 5 lymphocyte cells
                    (g/l): 0.15–0.40 protein
                    (%): 60 blood sugar

Abnormal test results

- ■ 10^3–10^4/mm polymorphs predominate, protein up to 3 and lowered blood sugar *suggests*:
  Bacterial infection

- ■ Up to 4000 cells, lymphocytes predominate, protein raised to 1–6, blood sugar 1.4 mmol/l *suggests*:
  TB

- ■ 10–20 000 cells/mm^3, lymphocytes present, protein up to 1.5, normal blood sugar *suggests*:
  Viral infection

NB CSF pressure = 70–180 mm of H$_2$O

Bacterial and viral causes of meningitis

Haemophilus influenza

Presentation

- Child < 5 years

Diagnosis

- Gram-negative Bacillus

Pneumococcus

Presentation

- Cranial nerve palsy, otitis media, lobar pneumonia
- Mortality 20%

Diagnosis

- Gram-positive, diplococcus, positive CSF, immunoelectropherosis

Mycobacterium tuberculosis

Presentation

- Subacute onset, Pyrexia of Unknown Origin (PUO), cranial nerve lesions
- Fits in children

Diagnosis

- Acid and alcohol fast bacilli on Ziehl-Neelsen staining

Coxsackie and echo virus

Presentation

- Paralysis (very rare)

Diagnosis

- Positive throat swab, positive stool culture, raised serum antibody titre

Mumps

Diagnosis

- Positive throat swab, positive stool culture, raised serum antibody titre

Poliovirus

Presentation

- Meningitis (common), asymmetrical paralysis (rare)

Diagnosis

- Positive throat swab, positive stool culture, raised serum antibody titre

FERTILITY AND PREGNANCY TESTING

FEMALE HORMONE PROFILES

- Measurement of female hormone levels (usually day 22 of the menstrual cycle) can indicate whether ovulation has occurred

Serum luteinising hormone (LH)

- Normal range (μmol/l): Follicular phase: 0.8–9.0
  Mid cycle: up to 65
  Luteal phase: 0.7–14.5

Serum follicle stimulating hormone (FSH)

- Normal range (μmol/l): Follicular phase: 1.5–11.5
  Mid cycle: up to 35
  Luteal phase: 0.7–8.5

Abnormal test result

- LH/FSH ratio > 3:1 *suggests*:
  Polycystic disease

Plasma progesterone

- Normal range (nmol/l): Follicular phase: 0.3–4.8
  Luteal phase: 7.9–8.9

Plasma oestradiol

- Normal range (pmol/l): Follicular phase: 40–170
  Mid cycle: 440–1400
  Luteal phase: 180–1000

Menopause

- Serum FSH and LH are both raised whilst the plasma oestradiol is lowered i.e. oestradiol 100–200 and FSH > 15–20

Serum prolactin

- Normal range (μg/l): Male: < 20
  Female in follicular phase: < 23
- Conditions causing raised levels of prolactin:
  Craniopharyngioma
  Myxoedema
  Renal failure
- Drugs causing raised levels of prolactin:
  Cimetidine
  Haloperidol
  Methyldopa
  Metoclopramide
  Oestrogens
  Phenothiazines

Abnormal test results

- Raised prolactin *may be a finding in*:
  Gynaecomastia
  Galactorrhoea
  Infertility
  Secondary amenorrhoea
  Impotence
  Dysfunctional bleeding

SEMEN ANALYSIS

- The initial investigation of male infertility
- The following are assessed:
  Total sperm count
  Sperm motility
  Volume of semen
- Normal range: Total count per ml: $50-200 \times 10^6$

  Motility: 90% after 45 min
  65% after 3 h

  Volume: 2–5 ml

  pH: 7.4
- Sperm morphology is of limited value in the assessment of infertility

PREGNANCY TESTS

- Urine pregnancy tests measure beta human chorionic gonadotrophin (HCG)
- First morning specimen should be tested; if unexpected negative result is obtained a random sample should be tested and checked against early morning sample
- Specimens should be stored in a refrigerator and tested within 72 h
- Assay of HCG usually positive in intrauterine pregnancy
- Assay of HCG only 50% positive in extrauterine, i.e. ectopic pregnancies
- Where an ectopic pregnancy is suspected the *blood* HCG should be requested, which is 200× more sensitive
- Patients who have repeated false-positive tests should have their serum HCG measured to check for chorion carcinoma

Pregnosticon

- Inhibition method standardised to detect 3.5 iu/ml of HCG
- Positive results can be expected 12 days *after* the first missed period or 40 days *after* the start of the last one

Abbott's Test Pack

- Monoclonal antibody enzyme immunoassay for the qualitative determination of HCG
- Positive results 4–5 days *before* a missed period

RHESUS BLOOD GROUP TESTING

- Incompatibilities in the rhesus blood group system between mother and child can result in the immunisation of the mother against her child, such that she produces antibodies that react to the fetal red cells, thereby causing haemolytic disease of the newborn (HDN)

All rhesus negative mothers

- With transfusions and/or obstetric history associated with HDN, samples required before 12th week, at 28th and 36th week and delivery
- With rhesus-positive infant: 6 month post-natal sample from mother
- With rhesus-negative infant: next pregnancy
- Rhesus-positive women with transfusion history require regular samples

Scheme for sampling pre- and postnatally

- Samples required before 12th week, at 28th and 36th weeks and at delivery:
  All known rhesus-negative women
  Rhesus-positive women who have a history of transfusion and/or an obstetric history associated with HDN since last tested
- Sample required 6 months postnatally:
  Rhesus-negative women delivered of a rhesus-positive infant
- Sample required at next pregnancy:
  Rhesus-negative women delivered of a rhesus-negative infant
- No further samples required:
  Rhesus-positive women with no transfusion or obstetric history
- Samples comprise 10 ml clotted blood and 5 ml blood for Hb

Kleihauer test

- All rhesus negative women should be tested within 24 h of a threatened miscarriage, miscarriage or termination of pregnancy (TOP)
- Fetal cells are looked for, dose of anti-D administered (250 or 500 iu within 72 h)

ALPHA FETO PROTEINS

Normal values in pregnancy (μg/l)

16 weeks gestation: 26.5 mean
                       < 10–53 range
                       > 64 neutral tube defect is likely
17 weeks gestation: 31 mean
                       < 10–62 range
                       > 74 neural tube defect is likely
18 weeks gestation: 34.5 mean
                       < 10–69 range
                       > 83 neural tube defect is likely

Abnormal test results

- Raised alpha feto proteins *suggests*:
  Open neural tube defects

- Lowered alpha feto proteins *may suggest*:
  Down's syndrome

Non-pregnant adults

Abnormal test results

- Alpha feto proteins > 500 μg/l *suggests*:
  Primary hepatoma

- Alpha feto proteins < 500 μg/l but > 40 g/l *suggests*:
  Primary or secondary hepatoma
  Cirrhosis
  Hepatitis
  Cancer in the GIT
  Cancer in the ovaries or testicles

MISCELLANEOUS

VIRILISM

Abnormal test results

- Plasma testosterone > 7 mmol/l, androstenedione sulphate > 35 mmol/l, 17-hydroxyprogesterone > 15 mmol/l *suggests*:
  Virilism
- Signs of virilism include:
  Bitemporal balding
  Clitoromegaly
  Deepening voice
  Hirsutism
  Male body build
- Organic causes of virilism:
  Adrenal tumours
  Congenital adrenal hyperplasia
  Cushing's syndrome
  Ovarian tumours

INTERPRETATION OF CERVICAL SMEARS

This is a guide to terms used by labs when reporting cervical smears. Different labs can use different terms; if there is any doubt over the meaning of a report or what action should be taken the individual lab should be consulted.

Inflammatory changes

- Probably best to ask lab exactly what is meant by this
- Cells probably show minimal changes, but not dyskaryosis or cytoplasmic changes

Action

- If there is vaginal discharge with identifiable cause treat before smear repeated
- Lab may recommend smear is repeated before the usual 3–5 years

Severe inflammatory changes

- Cellular changes may be progressive
- Vaginal discharge may mask abnormal cells

Action

- Follow-up required in 6 months or when lab recommends
- If 2 consecutive reports show these changes patient should be referred for colposcopy

Mild dyskaryosis, mild dysplasia or CIN 1

- Changes seen in CIN 1 may revert to normal

Action

- Colposcopy advisable
- Follow up as advised

Moderate dyskaryosis, moderate dysplasia or CIN 2

Action

- Colposcopy is mandatory

Severe dyskaryosis, severe dysplasia, CIN 3 or carcinoma *in situ*

Action

- Colposcopy is mandatory

Koilocytes

- Cells with a halo around their nucleus
- Indicates infection with human papilloma virus which causes genital warts
- Human papilloma virus may be involved in the aetiology of CIN

Action

- Cervical smears should be performed annually
- Could refer woman for colposcopy

Dyskeratosis

- Cornification/keratinisation of cells
- Indicates infection with human papilloma virus

Action

- Cervical smears should be performed annually
- Could refer woman for colposcopy

No endocervical cells seen

- Cells from the transformation area between squamous and columnar cells are absent (which is where most cervical cancers begin)
- Absence of these cells raises doubts over validity of smear

Action

- Some recommend repeat smear[5]

Postnatal smear

- Many polymorphs may be present and obscure cells such that abnormal cells cannot be excluded
- May be affected by altered hormonal state

Action

- Smear should be repeated

MICROSCOPIC HAEMATURIA

- Normal rate of urinary excretion of RBC: 20 000–40 000/h
  $$= < 200\,000 \text{ cells/ml}$$
- It is not uncommon for asymptomatic individuals to be detected on medical screening[6]

Abnormal test results

- Red cell count $> 100 \times 10^6/l$ in a centrifuged specimen *indicates*: Significant microscopic haematuria

Diagnosis

- Microscopy of unspun specimen of urine is unreliable;[7] it fails to reveal 80% of patients with known disease
- Centrifugation of urine increases sensitivity $\times 300$
- Urine Dipstix become positive at 50 000 cells/ml
- Commonest non-renal tract causes of false-positive Dipstix test:
  Menstruation in women
  Preputial or meatal lesions in men
  Following rectal examination
- Bacterial contamination or sterilisation of the urine bottle can give false-positive result on Dipstix
- Presence of RBC on microscopy, after centrifugation of urine, *confirms* haematuria and *excludes* false-positive Dipstix test
- Concurrent treatment with anticoagulants *does not exclude* renal tract pathology; investigation of microscopic haematuria should still be performed

Adult > 40 years

- Positive microscopy requires mid-stream urine specimen (MSU), cytoscopy and intravenous pyelogram (IVP)
- 20% will have substantial lesion of urinary tract and half of these a malignancy[8,9]
- Of those with no detectable abnormality a small proportion will develop a lesion over the next 3 years
- Concurrent treatment with anticoagulants *does not exclude* renal tract pathology and microscopic haematuria should still be investigated

Adult < 40 years

- Investigations probably do not require cytoscopy since malignancy is rare
- Haematuria associated with sport rarely lasts > 48 hr[10]
- Glomerulonephritis in the absence of proteinuria and hypertension is unlikely to be clinically significant and renal biopsy is rarely necessary
- The absence of any positive findings on investigation is known as benign or essential haematuria

Children

- Most common causes are glomerulonephritis, sickle cell disease and urinary tract infection
- Refer to paediatrician[11]

FAECAL FATS

- Normal range (mmol/24 h): Adult: 5–18
                              Children > 6 years: < 14

Test results

- Raised levels *suggests*:
  Malabsorption
  Pancreatic disease

Faecal Occult blood

Test results

- Positive *suggests*:
  Ulcerative and neoplastic disease of GIT

- Negative *suggests*:
  Does not *exclude* GIT disease
NB Contaminants from haemorrhoids and urethral blood may cause
a false-positive result

Reducing substances

- Presence in faeces *suggests* malabsorption e.g. lactase intolerance

THERAPEUTIC TARGET RANGES OF COMMONLY MONITORED DRUGS

- Check local lab ranges

	Metric units	Molar units
Aminophylline	10–15 µg/ml	
Carbamazepine	4–10 mg/l	17–42 µmol/l
Clonazepam	15–60 µg/l	
Digoxin	0.8–2.0 ng/l	1.0–2.6 nmol/l
Ethosuxamide	40–100 mg/l	283–708 µmol/l
Isoniazid	1–7 mg/l	
Lithium	4–11 mg/l	0.4–0.8 mmol/l
Phenobarbitone	10–40 mg/l	40–172 µmol/l
Phenytoin	10–20 mg/l	40–80 µmol/l
Primidone	5–12 mg/l	23–55 µmol/l
Sodium valproate	50–100 mg/l	347–693 µmol/l
Theophylline	10–20 mg/l	56–111 µmol/l

Lithium carbonate

- Therapeutic range (mmol/l): 0.4–0.8 12 h post-ingestion

Precautions

- Plasma concentrations must be measured regularly (every month on stabilised regimens)
- Thyroid function must be checked regularly and adequate sodium and fluid intake maintained

Possible contraindications

- Avoid in renal impairment, cardiac disease, conditions with sodium imbalance e.g. Addison's disease
- Caution in pregnancy (fetal intoxication), breast feeding mothers, elderly patients, myasthenia gravis and diuretic treatment

Dosage

- Initially 0.25–2.0 g daily

- Adjust to achieve plasma concentration of 0.4–0.8 mmol/l by tests on samples taken 12 h after the preceding dose on the 4th and 7th days of treatment, then weekly until dosage has remained constant for 4 weeks and monthly thereafter
- Daily doses are usually divided and sustained-release preparations are normally given 2× daily
- Dose adjustment may be necessary in diarrhoea, vomiting and heavy sweating

Overdosage

- The following *will* occur with severe Li^+ overdose i.e. plasma concentration > 2 mmol/l:
  Hyper-reflexia
  Hyperextension of limbs
  Convulsions
  Toxic psychoses
  Syncope
  Oliguria
  Circulatory failure
  Coma
- The following *may* occur with severe Li^+ overdose:
  Goitre
  Raised antidiuretic hormone concentration
  Hypothyroidism
  Hypokalaemia
  ECG changes
  Exacerbation of psoriasis
  Kidney changes
  Death

Side effects

- Short term:
  Diarrhoea
  Fine tremor
  Indigestion
  Nausea
  Polydypsia
  Polyuria

- Long term:
  The above *plus*:
  Exacerbation of psoriasis
  Hypothyroidism
  Memory loss
  Weight gain

Drugs affecting lithium levels

- Drugs that increase plasma lithium:
  Phenylbutazone and possibly other NSAIDs
  Thiazide diuretics e.g. bendrofluazide (Aprinox, Centyl, Neo-Naclex), chlorthalidone (Hygroton), xipamide (Diurexan) and indapamide (Natrilix)
  Other potassium-sparing diuretics e.g. triamterene (Dytac) do not have any effect on serum lithium
  Since Ibuprofen is available OTC, patients should be warned of the possible adverse effects; aspirin has no such effect
- Drugs that decrease plasma lithium:
  Theophylline
  Acetazolamide
  Sandocal
  Fybogel
  Some antacids e.g. sodium bicarbonate, magnesium trisilicate (Gaviscon)

NB Cessation of Li$^+$ therapy 2–3 days before elective surgery should be considered although the risk of precipitating a psychotic relapse should be weighed against the benefits

IMMUNOFLUORESCENT AUTOANTIBODIES

Antinuclear antibodies (ANA)

Test results

- Titre < 1:40
  Of doubtful significance

- Titre > 1:80
  Can be significant particularly in children and men but weak positive results are quite common in women > 40 years

- Titre ≥ 1:160
  Requires further immunological investigation

- Positive ANA *suggests*:
  Connective tissue disease
  Liver problems
  Some autoimmune lung diseases

- Negative ANA largely *excludes* lupus especially if there is no skin involvement

Thyroid antibodies

Test results

- Titre > 1:40
  Check thyroid function tests every 2 years as hypothyroidism in this group is significantly increased
  See also p. 35–7

Parietal cell antibodies

Test results

- Positive *may suggest*:
  PA
  Check MCV and B_{12} levels
  Consider intrinsic factor antibody testing

Rheumatoid factors

- Rheumatoid arthritis haemagglutination assay (RAHA) test has replaced the Rose Waaler test for RA in many labs
- RAHA titre 1:80 = Rose Waaler (SCAT/DAT) 1:16
- RAHA test is positive in 80% of rheumatoid patients
- There is a false-positive rate of 5% in normal population

Test results

■ Titre 1:80 = weak positive

■ Titre 1:160 = significant

Differential diagnosis

- If a patient suspected of having RA is seronegative (i.e. negative RAHA) obtain help from X-rays where RA may be distinguished from psoriasis and oesteoarthritis (OA) once disease has been present for 1–2 years
- Rheumatoid factors can be found less frequently in other connective tissue diseases, e.g. lupus, chronic infective endocarditis and tuberculosis, usually at lower levels

Smooth muscle antibodies

Test results

■ Positive *suggests*:
Liver disease
Transient viral infections

Antimitochondrial antibodies

Test results

■ Positive *suggests*:
Primary biliary cirrhosis
Perform LFT
- Early referral to liver specialist may be required

Reticulin antibodies

Test results

■ Positive *suggests*:
Small bowel disease in particular coeliac problems

Antiribosomal antibodies

● A rare serological presentation of lupus

DNA Antibody

● Occurs in connective tissue disorders and may help to distinguish drug induced disorders e.g. drug induced lupus

Corioembryonic antigen (CEA)

● Occurs in metastatic disease and colorectal cancer
● Normal range (mg/ml): < 3

Abnormal test results

■ > 20 *suggests*:
Repeat test after 1 month

■ > 35 *suggests*:
Metastatic carcinoma

■ > 100 *suggests*:
Probable hepatic metastasis

NB 3–10 *may occur in*:
Heavy smokers
Chronic lung disease
Cirrhosis
Pancreatitis
Inflammatory bowel disease
Peptic ulcers
Renal failure

Complement

Normal range (g/l): Plasma C_3: 0.63–1.19
  Plasma C_4: 0.11–0.43

Test results

■ Low C_3 and/or C_4 *suggests*:
  Complement activation

C_3 degradation products (iu/ml)

● Slight elevation: 13–15
● Moderate elevation: 16–20
● Gross elevation: > 20

C-reactive protein (CRP)

● Useful test to monitor activity of RA
● Normal range (mg/l): 0–8
● May be positive in malignancy when ESR remains normal

BODY MASS INDEX (BMI)

- Useful guide to the most appropriate mass of an individual as opposed to weight alone
- To calculate divide weight in kg by height in m
- Normal range (kg/m^2): Male: 20–25
- Female: 18.5–23

RECOMMENDED WEIGHTS, ADAPTED FROM DATA FROM THE FOGARTY CONFERENCE, USA, 1979 AND THE ROYAL COLLEGE OF PHYSICIANS 1981

Height without shoes (m)	Weight range recommended without clothes (kg)		Weight at BMI 27
	Men	Women	
1.45		42–53	57
1.48		42–54	59
1.50		43–55	61
1.52		44–57	62
1.54		44–58	64
1.56		45–58	66
1.58	51–64	46–59	67
1.60	52–65	48–61	69
1.62	53–66	49–62	71
1.64	54–67	50–64	73
1.66	55–69	51–65	74
1.68	56–71	52–66	76
1.70	58–73	53–67	78
1.72	59–74	55–69	80
1.74	60–75	56–70	82
1.76	62–77	58–72	84
1.78	64–79	59–74	86
1.80	65–80		87
1.82	66–82		89
1.84	67–84		91
1.86	69–86		93
1.88	71–88		95
1.90	73–90		97
1.92	75–93		99

PEAK FLOW RATE (l/min) IN ADULT MALES

	20	25	30	35	40	45	50	55	Age (years)
Height (cm) 157.48	124	126	130	132	135	137	138	139	
160.02	125	129	133	135	138	140	141	142	
162.56	128	133	136	138	141	143	144	145	
165.10	133	137	140	142	145	147	148	149	
167.64	138	141	144	146	149	151	152	153	
170.18	141	145	148	150	153	155	156	158	
172.72	145	149	152	155	158	160	161	163	
175.26	149	153	156	160	163	165	166	168	
177.80	153	157	161	165	168	170	171	173	
180.34	158	162	166	170	174	176	177	178	
182.88	162	167	172	176	180	182	183	184	
185.42	169	173	178	182	186	188	190	191	
187.96	175	179	184	189	193	195	197	198	

PEAK FLOW RATE (l/min) IN ADULT FEMALES

	20	25	30	35	40	45	50	55	Age (years)
Height (cm) 147.32	110	113	116	119	123	126	129	129	
149.86	112	115	118	121	125	128	131	131	
152.40	113	117	120	123	127	130	133	133	
154.94	116	119	122	125	129	132	135	135	
157.48	118	121	124	127	132	135	138	138	
160.02	121	124	127	130	135	138	141	141	
162.56	125	128	131	134	138	141	144	144	
165.10	128	131	135	138	142	145	148	148	
167.64	132	135	139	142	146	149	152	152	
170.18	136	139	142	146	150	153	156	158	
172.72	140	143	146	150	154	157	161	163	
175.26	144	147	150	154	158	161	165	167	
177.80	148	151	154	157	161	164	169	171	

REFERENCES

1 Penn R & Worthington DJ (1983). Is serum gamma glutamyl transferase a misleading test? *BMJ* **286**: 531–5

2 Coronary heart disease, the need for action. Office of Health Economics, 1987 No. 86

3 Ball M & Mann J (1988). Lipids and heart disease, a practical approach. OUP

4 Goh BT (1987). Sexually transmitted diseases. *Prescriber's Journal* **275**: 18–29

5 Alexander I (1988). Chlamydia, one step forward, two steps back. *BMJ* **297**: 791

6 Ritchie CD, Bevan EA & Collier STJ (1986). Importance of occult haematuria found at screening. *BMJ* **292**: 681–3

7 Kesson AM, Talbot SM & Gyory AZ (1978). Microscopic examination of urine. *Lancet* **ii**: 809–12

8 Carson CC, Segura JW & Green LF (1978). Clinical importance of micro-haematuria. *JAMA* **241**: 149–50

9 Golin AL & Howard RS (1980). Asymptomatic microscopic haematuria. *J Urol* **124**: 389–91

10 Siegal AJ, Hennekans CH, Solomans HS & Van Boekal B (1979). Exercise related haematuria. Findings in a group of marathon runners. *JAMA* **241**: 391–2

11 Bullock B (1986). Asymptomatic microscopical haematuria. *BMJ* **292**: 645

INDEX

Abbott's test pack   67
actinomyces-like organisms   53–4
activated partial thromboplastin
    time   12
acute aseptic meningitis   60
agranulocytosis   8
alanine aminotransferase   16–17
albumin   18
alcohol
    abuse   21–2
    intoxication   22
alkaline phosphatase   15–16, 18
ALO   53–4
alpha feto protein   69
alpha-globulins   18–19
ALT   16–17
aminophylline, therapeutic target
    range   77
ANA   80
anaemia   3–6
androstenedione sulphate, plasma
    levels in females   70
anisocytes   14
antimitochondrial antibodies   81
antinuclear antibodies (ANA)   80
antiribosomal antibodies   82
aplastic anaemia   4
ascaris   48–9
aspartate aminotransferase (AST)
    16–17
AST   16–17

basophils   7–8
Bence Jones protein   20
beta-globulins   18–19
bicarbonate, serum   23
bile pigments, urinary   15
bilirubin
    serum   15
    urinary   15
bleeding time   11
blood coagulation tests   11–13
blood group testing   67

blood lipids   38–45
blood sugar   30–2
BMI   84
body mass index (BMI)   84
bone disease, differential diagnosis
    29
Branhamella catarrhalis   57

C-reactive protein   83
C_3 degradation products   83
calcium   28
    excretion over 24 hours   27
Campylobacter jejuni   47–8
Campylobacter pylori   48
carbamazepine, therapeutic target
    range   77
carcinoma in situ   72
CEA   82–3
cerebrospinal fluid   60–3
cervical smears, interpretation   71–3
chlamydia   52–3
chloride
    excretion over 24 hours   27
    serum   23
cholesterol   38–45
chronic lymphatic leukaemia (CLL)
    8
CK   33
CLL   8
clonazepam, therapeutic target
    range   77
clotting time   11
complement   83
complement fixation tests   51
copper, serum   23
corioembryonic antigen   82–3
cortisol, serum   23
Coxsackie and echo virus   62
creatine excretion over 24 hours   27
creatine kinase   33
creatinine
    excretion over 24 hours   27
    serum   23
CRP   83

cryptosporidia 48

diabetes mellitus
confirmation of 30
monitoring long-term control
31–2
diarrhoea, infectious 46–8
differential white blood-cell count
7–8
digoxin, therapeutic target range 77
DNA antibody 82
drugs, therapeutic target ranges 77
Duke's bleeding time 11
dysbetalipoproteinaemia, familial
42–3
dyskariosis 71–2
dyskeratosis 72
dysplasia, cervical 71–2

electrolytes 23–5
Enterobius vermicularis 49
eosinophils 7–8
erythrocyte sedimentation rate
(ESR) 9
ESR 9
ethanol concentrations 22
ethosuxamide, therapeutic target
range 77

faecal fats 76
faecal occult blood 76
familial combined hyperlipidaemia
42
familial dysbetalipoproteinaemia
42–3
familial hypercholesterolaemia 41
familial triglyceridaemia 42
fats, faecal 76
FDP 12
female hormone profiles 64–5
fertility testing 64–5
fibrin degradation products (FDP)
12
fibrinogen, plasma 11–12
folate 6
follicle stimulating hormone, serum
(FSH) 64
free thyroxine index 35
fructosamine, serum 32
FSH, serum 64

FT$_4$I 35

gamma-globulins 18–20
gamma glutamyl transferase (GGT)
16, 17–18
Gardnerella vaginalis 52
gastrointestinal organisms 46–9
GGT 16, 17–18
Giardia lamblia 47
globulins 18–19
glucose tolerance test (GTT) 30–1
gonorrhoea 50–1
Graves' disease 36, 37
GTT 30–1

haemagglutination test for thyroid
antibodies 36–7
haematocrit 1
haematuria, microscopic 74–5
haemoglobin 1
haemolysis 3
Haemophilus influenza 61
Haemophilus vaginalis 52
haptoglobin 6
Hb 1
HbA$_1$ 31–2
HCG 66
Herpes genitalis 50
hormone profiles, female 64
homovanillic acid (HVA) 26, 28
human chorionic gonadotrophin 66
HVA 26, 28
17-hydroxyprogesterone, plasma
levels in females 70
hypercalcaemia 28
hypercholesterolaemia, principles of
treatment of 39–41
familial 41
hyperglycaemia, causes of 31
hyperlipidaemia, familial combined
42
hyperlipoproteinaemia 39–43
classification 43–4
management 44
hyperparathyroidism 29, 36
hyperthyroidism 35–6
hyperuricaemia 24–5
hypocalcaemia 28
hypochromasia 14
hypochromic microcytic anaemia 3

hypoglycaemia, causes of   31
hypothyroidism   29, 36

IgA   19–20
IgG   19–20
IgM   19–20
immunofluorescent autoantibodies
     80–3
immunoglobulins   19–20
infertility testing   64–5
INR   13
international normalised ratio
     (INR)   13
isoniazid, therapeutic target range
     77

jaundice   17, 20–1

kaolin cephalic clotting time
     (KCCT)   12
KCCT   12
Kleihauer test   68
koilocytes   72

lactic dehydrogenase   34
large unstained cells (LUC)   8
LDH   34
lead, serum   23
leucocytosis   7–8
leucopenia   8
leukaemia, chronic lymphatic   8
LFT   15–22
LH, serum   64
lipid disorders, rare   41–3
lipoproteins   38–45
lithium carbonate   77–9
liver function tests (LFT)   15–22
Loeffler's syndrome   48
LUC   8
luteinising hormone, serum (LH)   64
lymphocytes   7–8

macrocytic anaemia   4
magnesium excretion over 24 hours
     27
MCH   2
MCHC   2
MCV   1, 17
mean corpuscular haemoglobin
     (MCH)   2

mean corpuscular haemoglobin
     concentration (MCHC)   2
mean corpuscular volume (MCV)   1,
     17
megaloblastic anaemia   4
meningitis   58, 60–3
meningococcal meningitis   58
menopause, hormone levels   64
metabolite excretion   27
microscopic haematuria   74–5
monocytes   7–8
mumps   62
Mycobacterium tuberculosis   62
myeloma   20
myxoedema   35–6

nematode   48–9
neural tube defects   68
neutrophils   7–8
nitrogen excretion over 24 hours   27
normochromic normocytic anaemia
     3
5-nucleotidase   16

occult blood, faecal   76
oestradiol, plasma   64
osmolality   28
osteomalacia   29
17 oxosteroids   17, 26
     excretion over 24 hours   27
17 oxygenic steroids   26

packed cell volume   1
Paget's disease   29
pancytopenia   4
parietal cell antibodies   80
PCV   1
peak flow rates   85–6
pernicious anaemia   6
phaeochromocytoma   28
phenobarbitone, therapeutic target
     range   77
phenytoin, therapeutic target range
     77
phosphate   29
     excretion over 24 hours   27
plasma fibrinogen   11–12
platelets   10
Pneumococcus   61–2
Pneumocystis carinii   57–8

poliomyelitis 60
Poliovirus 63
polycythaemia rubra vera 1, 5
postnatal smear 73
potassium
  disturbances 23–4
  excretion over 24 hours 27
  serum 23
pregnancy tests 67
Pregnosticon 67
primidone, therapeutic target range
  77
progesterone, plasma 64
prolactin, serum 65
protein
  excretion over 24 hours 27
  serum 18–20
prothrombin ratio 13
prothrombin time 12
PRV 1, 5
pseudopolycythaemia 1, 5
pyogenic meningitis 60

RBC 2
red blood-cell count (RBC) 2
red cell folate 6
red cell indices 1–2
reducing substances 76
reticulin antibodies 82
rhesus blood group testing 68
rheumatoid factors 81
rickets 29

salmonella 46
sampling, blood lipids 39
semen analysis 66
serum bilirubin 15
serum electrolytes 23–5
serum ferritin 4–5
serum folate 6
serum free T$_3$ 35
serum free T$_4$ 35
serum fructosamine 31–2
serum haptoglobin 6
serum iron 5
serum prolactin 65
serum proteins 18–20
shigella 46–7
Simplate II technique 11
skin bleeding times 11

smooth muscle antibodies 81
sodium
  disturbances 23
  excretion over 24 hours 27
  serum 23
sodium valproate, therapeutic target
  range 77
spherocytes 14
streptococcus 58
stress polycythaemia 1, 5
subarachnoid haemorrhage 60
sugar, blood 30–2
syphilis 54–5

T$_3$ 35–6
T$_4$ 35–6
target cells 14
TBG 35–6
testosterone, plasma levels in
  females 70
theophylline, therapeutic target
  range 77
threadworm 49
thrombin time 13
thrombo test 13
thrombophilia 13
thyroid antibodies 36–7, 80
thyroid function tests 35–7
thyroid releasing hormone (TRH)
  stimulation test 36
thyroid stimulating hormone (TSH)
  35–6
thyrotoxicosis 35–6
thyrotrophin antibody test (TRAb)
  36
thyroxine binding globulin (TBG)
  35–6
TIBC 5
total iron binding capacity (TIBC) 5
total thyroxine (T$_4$) 35–6
toxoplasma 56–7
TRAb test 36
TRH stimulation test 36
Trichomonas vaginalis 51–2
triglyceridaemia, familial 42
tri-iodothyronine (T$_3$) 35–6
TSH 35–6
tuberculosis 61
tuberculous meningitis 60

urate   24–5
   excretion over 24 hours   27
urea
   excretion over 24 hours   27
   serum   23
urinary bile pigments   15
urinary tract infection (UTI)   59
urine biochemistry   26–9
urobilinogen   15
urogenital organisms   50–5
UTI   59

vanilmandelic acid (VMA)   26

virilism   70
vitamin B_{12} 6
VMA   26

warfarin therapy, effects on test
      results   13
WBC   7
white blood cell count (WBC)   7–9
white cell indices   7–9
whole blood clotting time   11
Widal test   46

zinc, serum   23